Rheumatoid Arthritis

How to Identify if You Have Rheumatoid Arthritis

(A Guide to the Natural Approach Against Rheumatoid Arthritis)

Michael McDonald

Published By **John Kembrey**

Michael McDonald

Rheumatoid Arthritis: How to Identify if You Have Rheumatoid Arthritis (A Guide to the Natural Approach Against Rheumatoid Arthritis)

ISBN **978-1-998038-08-4**

Legal & Disclaimer

Table Of Contents

Chapter 1: Rheumatoid Arthritis Overview
.... 1

Chapter 2: Complications & Comorbidities
In Rheumatoid Arthritis 11

Chapter 3: Sexual Health In Rheumatoid
Arthritis.. 21

Chapter 4: Rheumatoid Arthritis During
Pregnancy & Lactation 25

Chapter 5: Course Of Rheumatoid Arthritis
.... 27

Chapter 6: Economic Burden Due To
Rheumatoid Arthritis 29

Chapter 7: Rheumatoid Arthritis Flare & Its
Management 33

Chapter 8: Emotional And Psychological
Aspects In Rheumatoid Arthritis And Its
Management 38

Chapter 9: Role Of Exercise, Joint
Protection Maneuvers & Activities Of Daily

Living In Patients With Rheumatoid Arthritis.................................. 51

Chapter 10: Diet Modifications And Maintaining Adequate Body Weight In Patients With Rheumatoid Arthritis 67

Chapter 11: Quality Of Life In Rheumatoid Arthritis & Ways To Improve It............... 83

Chapter 12: Real Life Scenarios Of Rheumatoid Arthritis Patients................ 89

Chapter 13: Importance Of Regular Visits To A Doctor 95

Chapter 14: Medicines To Treat Rheumatoid Arthritis Patients................ 97

Chapter 15: Blueprint To A Pain Free Life Amongst Patients With Rheumatoid Arthritis.. 113

Chapter 16: Background To Rheumatoid Arthritis.. 117

Chapter 17: Risk Factors And The Search For Possible Causes............................. 137

Chapter 18: Glucocorticoids................. 151

Chapter 19 : Abatacept (Orencia®)....... 171

Chapter 1: Rheumatoid Arthritis Overview

WHAT IS RHEUMATOID ARTHRITIS?

Rheumatoid arthritis (RA) is an autoimmune disorder in which the affected character's immune device mistakenly attacks its very non-public frame questioning as remote places. It is a persistent inflammatory disorder which could have an effect on joints and unique organs of the frame like coronary heart, brain, kidneys, lungs, eyes, and masses of others. RA is the most commonplace inflammatory joint illness, visible in 1-2% of the populace round the arena. The contamination associated with rheumatoid arthritis can have an effect on fundamental organs of the frame like pores and pores and skin, eyes, lungs, coronary heart, kidneys, nerves and blood vessels. With the advent of recent drug treatments, a affected individual with rheumatoid arthritis stands a brilliant threat to live a normal to close to normal lifestyles.

1

RISK FACTORS OF RHEUMATOID ARTHRITIS

Factors which increase risk of growing RA are -

1.Age - RA can start at any age, though generally it takes region in center age.

2. Sex - RA typically impacts girls, -to-3 instances better than men.

3.Genes - People whose frame incorporate unique genes along with HLA (human leukocyte antigen) are much more likely to expand RA.

4.Family History – Those with a family statistics of RA are at expanded threat of growing the same. The hazard isn't always 100 %, however a small growth as compared to the general populace.

5.Smoking – Smoking is an established hazard factor for RA. Smoking makes the illness worse and increases chance of lung development in RA.

6.Obesity - Being obese will increase the risk of growing RA

7.Environment – Chemical exposure or certain viral infections boom the hazard of growing RA

8.Diet - Drinking sugary soda on a ordinary foundation will increase the danger of growing rheumatoid arthritis

Taking care of dental hygiene permits manage infection related to rheumatoid arthritis. Thus, correct dental health can help manage RA.

SYMPTOMS OF RHEUMATOID ARTHRITIS –

Rheumatoid arthritis ought to have numerous manifestations. Its manifestations define the symptoms which a affected individual can boom. Common signs and signs and symptoms of RA encompass:

•Pain, stiffness or swelling in a single or more joint

•Weight loss

•Fever

•Fatigue, inclined element or tiredness

Symptoms also can range depending on the organ worried. For instance – a affected person might also additionally have pink eyes, dryness in the eyes (gritty feeling), dry mouth, dry pores and pores and skin, dry cough, rashes over pores and pores and skin and so forth.

HOW IS RHEUMATOID ARTHRITIS DIAGNOSED?

RA is a scientific diagnosis, identified with the beneficial resource of regular symptoms and signs and symptoms and signs and symptoms after analyzing a affected man or woman with supportive proof from lab tests. Tests like ESR and CRP can be raised in sufferers with RA, mainly at the time of disease hobby. Rheumatoid hassle and/or anti CCP ranges are normally raised in patients with RA, however may be in regular range in 30-forty percentage sufferers. So, a terrible

Rheumatoid element or anti CCP levels does no longer rule out its analysis.

RHEUMATOID ARTHRITIS – WHICH ALL ORGANS CAN IT INVOLVE?

Rheumatoid arthritis may also have extra articular (involvement other than joints) manifestations in about 40% of patients. These manifestations can rise up either in the beginning or each time all through the route in their contamination.

Cimmino MA, Salvarani C, Macchioni P. Extra-articular manifestations in 587 Italian sufferers with rheumatoid arthritis. Rheumatol Int. 2000;19(6):213–217.

These manifestations are greater common in sufferers with energetic and extreme RA. Thus, early competitive approach shall seem like suitable in view of the terrible effect of more articular manifestations on RA consequences. Rheumatoid arthritis is related to a excessive hazard of morbidity and premature loss of existence secondary to the earlier improvement of cardiovascular, lung illnesses and malignancy.

Crostein BN. Interleukin-6 – a key mediator of systemic and nearby signs and symptoms in rheumatoid arthritis. Bull NYU Hosp J Dis. 2007;sixty 5(Suppl 1): S11–S15.

Extra articular involvement in RA includes –

1. Skin

2. Eyes

3. Mouth (oral)

four. Lungs

five. Cardiac (coronary coronary heart)

6. Kidneys

7. Neurological

eight. Hematological (blood)

SKIN INVOLVEMENT

Rheumatoid nodules (lumps over bone or pores and skin) are the most not unusual pores and pores and skin manifestations in RA. They are seen in spherical 20% of sufferers with RA. Rheumatoid vasculitis (swelling of blood vessels) can be visible at the pores and pores and skin. It can also seem within the shape of haemorrhages (crimson spots on pores and pores and skin), ulcers over the leg and gangrene of fingers. The patient may additionally additionally have dry pores and pores and skin due to the truth the manifestation due to the secondary sjogren syndrome.

EYE INVOLVEMENT

The most common eye manifestation is dry eyes seen in spherical 10-15% sufferers with RA. Sometimes, it could be the primary manifestation of RA. Other manifestations of eyes in RA encompass – pink eyes, which can be painless or painful. Rarely, ulcers can amplify within the eyes, that might result in corneal melt.

ORAL MANIFESTATIONS

Dry mouth can be a manifestation of patients with RA. Decreased manufacturing of saliva can bring about dental caries. Patients with RA who increase dental caries have aggressive disorder, hard to govern with drug remedies. A proper treatment of dental caries can remedy this trouble.

LUNG MANIFESTATION

Lung involvement can also arise within the shape of interstitial lung disease which might also furthermore occur as a dry cough. Patients with RA have accelerated hazard of being asthmatics which may additionally additionally take region as wheezing, breathing problem with or without cough. There may be nodules in the lungs. Patients with RA are at immoderate hazard of acquiring lung infections as pneumonia, tuberculosis, and so on.

CARDIAC DISEASE

The chance for coronary heart attack in lady sufferers with RA isinstances that of a everyday healthful lady. In long-standing disease of at least 10 years, the chance of heart attack is 3 times better as compared to the overall populace. Patients with RA greater regularly increase coronary coronary heart failure than human beings with ordinary healthy populations. Heart involvement in RA will increase the hazard of premature demise.

KIDNEY INVOLVEMENT

Kidney involvement in RA is unusual. Rarely, infection within the kidneys can purpose protein leakage.

NEUROLOGICAL MANIFESTATIONS

Nerve involvement is not unusual in RA sufferers. The affected person also can experience numbness, burning, paresthesias, weak point of palms or ft. When a nerve of hand (median nerve) is affected, it's far referred to as carpal tunnel syndrome. It may also moreover seem as involvement of a joint some of the cranium and spinal wire which, if excessive, can bring about paralysis.

HEMATOLOGICAL (BLOOD) INVOLVEMENT

RA may also moreover moreover bring about low haemoglobin, growth in platelets and coffee leukocyte depend huge range. RA will increase the threat of blood cancers as lymphoma or leukemia.

PSYCHIATRIC MANIFESTATIONS

RA is associated with psychosomatic manifestations as anxiety and depression. Depression and anxiety in RA patients have poor remedy outcomes.

Chapter 2: Complications & Comorbidities In Rheumatoid Arthritis

Untreated, prolonged status or improperly controlled rheumatoid arthritis patients are positive to increase complications and comorbidities. The identical might also additionally expand in managed contamination further to in early disorder but the percentage is a fantastic deal lots lots much less in such times.

COMPLICATIONS IN RHEUMATOID ARTHRITIS

Most of the sufferers anticipate that rheumatoid arthritis is a sickness of the joints. As described earlier, it may have an effect on many organ systems in the body. Just like swelling/contamination in the joints, RA can purpose infection in critical organs of the frame for this reason most important to harm and RA related complications. RA related complications are -

1.Joint Damage –

Rheumatoid arthritis if not handled early or now not properly controlled can bring about joint damage, which also can require surgical treatment. Inflammation or joint swelling can harm the joint cartilage, tendons and close by bone. This may also moreover bring about joint deformities and disabilities.

2.Osteoporosis-

Osteoporosis method prone bones for that reason important to increase in threat of fracture. Osteoporosis in RA is majorly because of Rheumatoid arthritis itself, at the aspect of some contribution from medicinal capsules used in its treatment. The lifetime hazard of developing fracture is as immoderate as 40% in sufferers who increase osteoporosis in RA.

three.Infections –

Patients with RA are at prolonged danger of mild to lifestyles threatening infections. The threat of contamination is maximum whilst the infection is lively. Risk of infection is contributed greater through the usage of the disorder interest then by using drug remedies used to address the sickness barring some infections. Vaccines are recommended to prevent infections in RA.

four.Abnormal body composition -

Patients of RA have better fat to lean mass ratio, even in humans who've a normal body mass index (BMI). Patients with RA lose muscle tissue but regain fat which predisposes the affected individual to cardiovascular sicknesses.

5.Heart problems –

Rheumatoid arthritis will boom the risk of hardening and blockage of arteries. Patients with RA have high hazard of growing cardiovascular disorder. There is expanded risk of having heart attack, stroke and coronary heart failure. Smoking, weight troubles, comorbidity like diabetes, deranged body ldl ldl cholesterol and improved blood pressure, horrible weight-reduction plan and insufficient exercising are hazard factors similarly to out of manage rheumatoid arthritis which in addition growth the danger of cardiovascular disease.

6.Lung disease –

People with rheumatoid arthritis have an stepped forward danger of infection and shrinkage of the lung. This can cause dry cough and modern shortness of breath. People with RA are at prolonged chance of growing lung infections as pneumonia, tuberculosis, and so forth.

7.Lymphoma -

Rheumatoid arthritis will increase the chance of blood most cancers as lymphoma. Some research component out that patients with RA have improved chance of growing lung, liver and esophageal maximum cancers.

8.Memory Loss, Anxiety & melancholy –

Memory loss, tension and melancholy are common in sufferers with rheumatoid arthritis seen in nearly1/3 of sufferers. Patients can also enjoy uneasiness, loss of sleep, palpitations, ghabrahat, horrible feelings or idea and forgetfulness. These manifestations might also result in skipping drug remedies and boom in pain.

IS RHEUMATOID ARTHRITIS CURABLE?

RA is a long time disorder requiring long term remedy, however this have to now not frighten the affected person. Just like high blood pressure, thyroid sicknesses, diabetes, coronary heart ailments and so on RA too require lifelong remedy. Just like excessive blood strain and diabetes, everyday remedy if commenced out early need to control the ailment and save you deformities and disabilities. Long time period research show that 10-14% of patients of early RA (disorder period much less than 2 years) skip into long time remission (absence of any signal & symptoms) with out drug treatments.

ARE RA PATIENTS AT RISK OF PREMATURE DEATH?

RA is on the complete considered a disorder of only joints with the aid of most humans. They assume that this sickness obtained't have an effect on their existence span as it handiest affects their joints. However, this isn't true. Inflammation takes region in every and each a part of the frame much like swelling inside the joints.

•Lifespan of an RA affected person is 10-15 years shorter than not unusual normal

• However, RA sufferers whose sickness were below manipulate - may additionally have ordinary existence expectancy

• Factors proven to reduce existence span – cardiovascular ailment, respiratory involvement as ILD, Obstructive airway disease, infections as pneumonia, musculoskeletal scenario as deformities

Complications that determines the existence span of sufferers with RA –

•how a long way RA has progressed

•sex, with women (threat of immoderate RA is extra)

•early prognosis and remedy associated with minimal complications and favorable consequences

•Individual threat elements, as a family statistics of coronary heart sickness, diabetes

•Smoking and eating alcohol had been related to decreased lifestyles span

•   Medications – sickness-editing antirheumaticdrugs (methotrexate, sulfasalazine, hydroxychloroquine, leflunomide) and biologics lessen the hazard of complications

•Early analysis and treatment - controls infection - reduces the danger of demise

COMORBIDITIES IN RHEUMATOID ARTHRITIS

Comorbidities in RA patients are improved compared to the general populace. Comorbidities growth in RA sufferers as RA reasons infection in all organs of the body from head to toe. On a mean, RA sufferers haveor more co morbid conditions.

Michaud K, Wolfe F. Comorbidities in rheumatoid arthritis. Best Pract Res Clin Rheumatol. 2007;21(5):885-906. Doi:10.1016/j.Berh.2007.06.002

These co morbid situations increase the threat of untimely demise in RA sufferers.

Dougados M, Soubrier M, Perrodeau E et al. Impact of a nurse-led programme on comorbidity control and impact of a affected character self-evaluation of ailment activity on the manage of rheumatoid arthritis: results of a capacity, multicentre, randomised, controlled trial (COMEDRA). Ann. Rheum. Dis. Seventy four(nine), 1725–1733 (2015).

Comorbidities related to RA are cardiovascular contamination (coronary coronary heart attack, paralysis or stroke), cancers (breast, blood, lung, pores and pores and skin and rectal); headaches related to infections (influenza, pneumonia), diabetes, elevated blood strain and deranged blood ldl cholesterol. Prevalence of comorbidities in patients with RA varies between 40 and sixty six%.

Daien. Assessment of comorbidities in rheumatoid arthritis. Revue. De. Medicine. Interne. forty, 40-43 (2019).

HOW TO REDUCE COMORBIDITIES IN RA

Dedicated and inspired sufferers always find it clean to govern RA and comorbidities.

Ways to lessen the comorbidities in RA are -

1. Control RA – Early control of RA alongside thing everyday test up with a rheumatologist reduces the risk of growing comorbidities.

2. Regular blood take a look at – Routine blood take a look at ordered with the aid of manner of your medical health practitioner goals to encounter any development of comorbidities. Detecting early and beginning drug treatments facilitates manage the

contamination, consequently stopping complications.

three. Weight loss – Weight loss in an obese or obese affected person reduces the hazard of development of comorbidity.

four. Diet control – Reducing chocolates, sugar, soda, soft liquids, fried meals and rapid meals allows lessen the danger of developing comorbidities in RA sufferers. If a affected individual with RA already has superior comorbidities, diet manipulate can assist reduce or manage the comorbidities.

5. Regular workout – Regular exercising not simplest controls RA signs and symptoms, however also lets in reduce the risk or controls comorbidities.

Chapter 3: Sexual Health In Rheumatoid Arthritis

Sexuality and its expression are crucial for healthful and unwell people and play an vital element in an individual's self-identification.

Sexual functioning is a neglected region of quality of life in sufferers with RA this is neither referred to with the aid of the usage of sufferers or scientific docs. RA might also additionally have an effect on all factors of life, along side sexual fitness. RA sufferers must experience faded sexual force because of frame and joint ache. The factors which have an impact on sexual functioning in RA are joint ache or stiffness, tiredness, beneficial impairment like deformities, depression, anxiety, terrible frame photo due to deformities, reduced desire for sex, hormonal imbalance and involvement of organs like coronary coronary heart, lungs. About 31-76% of arthritis sufferers revel in sexual troubles.

1. Gordon D, Beastall GH, Thomson JA, Sturrock RD. Androgenic popularity and sexual characteristic in guys with rheumatoid arthritis and ankylosing spondylitis. Q J Med 1986; 60: 671-679 [PMID: 3094090]

2. Kraaimaat FW, Bakker AH, Janssen E, Bijlsma JW. Intrusiveness of rheumatoid arthritis on sexuality in male and woman sufferers dwelling with a partner. Arthritis Care Res 1996; 9: a hundred and twenty-100 twenty 5 [PMID: 8970270]

Sexual function disturbances can stand up in advance than, at some point of and after sexual sports. Thus RA may have an effect on sexual health in a negative way. Manifestations of sexual incapacity encompass - trouble in assuming positive positions due to arthritis of hip or knee joint limiting actions, painful sex because of vaginal dryness and fatigue inside the route of intercourse.

Below is a tablet that suggests sexual sickness in RA patients, what factors cause such disorder and the way sufferers can enhance the sexual features. Patients ought talk about their sexual health with their doctor and might find out answers for the equal.

Sl. No.

Sexual sickness

Factors

Recommendations for sufferers

1

Sexual incapacity

Limited mobility, pain, fatigue, morning stiffness

Change characteristic, analgesic consumption, warm temperature and muscle rest earlier than hobby

2

Painful intercourse

Vaginal dryness

Vaginal lubrication, estrogen cream

three

Decreased choice

Anxiety, depression

Counselling, antidepressant capsules after consulting a physician.

Chapter 4: Rheumatoid Arthritis During Pregnancy & Lactation

Rheumatoid arthritis is a sickness that would have an effect on more youthful women of reproductive age institution. Due to this age organization, being pregnant and lactation aremost essential ranges wherein this illness could make an impact in a lady's existence. Controlling rheumatoid arthritis is the maximum vital hassle earlier than a affected person plans pregnancy. During pregnancy, RA gets subdued in maximum of the patients. However, in some it may get flared up. RA gets flared up located up shipping in maximum of the sufferers.

Medicines used to address RA need to be modified throughout pregnancy and lactation. All tablets aren't secure in the course of the ones unique times. There are many medicines which want to be stopped properly in advance in advance than making plans being pregnant. A affected man or woman want to consult his/her physician in advance than planning being pregnant, at some point of pregnancy and lactation on a ordinary foundation. Patients can also moreover require a few supplements within the route of being pregnant and lactation, which will be remarkable replied by way of way of manner of the treating clinical health practitioner.

Chapter 5: Course Of Rheumatoid Arthritis

Rheumatoid arthritis is a complex ailment. Its herbal route is variable in sufferers. For a few it could be a slight sickness not often requiring drug remedies. However, for a few it is able to be a nightmare because the infection may be so intense which hardly ever responds to any medicines. Course of RA varies from affected man or woman to affected person and is defined under -

•According to research, RA may also moreover get cured in 10-14% of sufferers, especially in those in which it is detected and treated early.

•15-20 percent of patients have intermittent disease with intervals of exacerbation and a fairly precise assessment.

•Some have periods of worsening symptoms and symptoms that trade with intervals of remission

•Most patients revel in, modern sickness (can also moreover progress slowly or speedy) and harm the bones, cartilage, and different systems of the joints

•Joint damage commonly worsens through the years and is irreversible and impact's person's normal sports, and result in massive disability

•RA can include primary organs of the frame like coronary heart, thoughts, kidney & lungs

•Deformities don't growth in often, but dealt with sufferers, however untreated or irregularly dealt with patients will increase deformities and require surgical procedures

•Regularly treated patients live everyday to close to everyday excellent of existence, but, it is negative in unusual or untreated patients

•Life expectancy is near normal in often handled patients but in untreated or irregular handled it's miles 15 years quick

Chapter 6: Economic Burden Due To Rheumatoid Arthritis

Rheumatoid arthritis not most effective impacts someone physical, but additionally drains him/her financially. It increases the economic burden to the diseased man or woman, however additionally to the family or maybe society. RA is associated with progressed comorbidities like diabetes, extended blood pressure, coronary coronary heart assaults, stroke and deranged ldl ldl ldl cholesterol. These comorbidities growth the economic burden amongst patients with RA. Studies concluded RA motives fantastic financial burden now not most effective for patients however as well the society. In advanced worldwide locations together with the united states, Canada and the UK, in which most of the direct charge is blanketed beneath coverage, art work-related disabilities and unwell leaves charge the economic machine a few billions of dollars. A have a have a observe stated that over a length of 10 years, arthritis associated paintings loss has been associated with a 37% drop in earnings. By assessment, human beings with out arthritis had a ninety% rise in income over the same period of time.

The monetary burden of RA sufferers is related to the direct and indirect costs of the disorder. Direct fees associated with rheumatoid arthritis is described through the technique applied in direct affected character care which includes –

1. Professional charge

2. Medication

3. Diagnostic

4. Hospitalization

five. Surgeries

6. Transportation

These prices are u . S . A . Precise, commonly being immoderate in superior global locations and coffee to mild in growing worldwide places.

Indirect charges don't forget the decreased earning functionality and decreased lifestyles expectancy. Indirect price is hard to estimate. Considering the age of onset of RA and disabilities related to it, indirect cost outweighs the direct price of RA.

Thus, RA substantially will increase the monetary burden among sufferers with RA.

WAYS TO DECREASE THE COST OF TREATMENT

Ways to reduce the rate are

1. Early remedy

2. Regular observe up

three. Regular exercise

four. Weight bargain

5. Controlling co-morbidities

Starting treatment early will save you deformities and disabilities and as a quit result prevent surgical procedures. Early treatment will manage illness early and received't require highly-priced capsules in most patients. Thus, a patient can resultseasily work at some point in their existence without affecting their expert life. This shall save you each direct and indirect charges.

Regular check up will help in early detection of any trouble be it because of disorder or drug remedies. Thus, an early intervention with the aid of the medical health practitioner will opposite the ones headaches consequently preventing hospitalisation and saving price.

Chapter 7: Rheumatoid Arthritis Flare & Its Management

DEFINITION

•Flares are intermittent bouts of improved rheumatoid arthritis ailment hobby causing fatigue, flu like symptoms and symptoms and signs and symptoms, pain, swelling and stiffness in joints

•Other signs and signs associated with it – sleep disturbance, generalized body ache, difficulty in doing day by day artwork

CAUSES OF RA FLARE

Some stated reasons are –

➢STRESS – Stress is a mentioned reason for plenty sicknesses and RA is not any exception.

➢INFECTIONS – as moderate as the common cold can boom RA sickness hobby.

➢ FOODS – Exact culprit is tough to pinpoint as complex meals is wonderful for one-of-a-kind sufferers. Patients can listing down food which doesn't wholesome them and should avoid the ones components.

➤ OVER EXERTION – Over exertion is related to an growth in RA contamination interest.

➤ POST DELIVERY - Pregnancy is associated with an altered immune system. Post-transport, the immune machine has a bent to head decrease lower back to everyday but from time to time it turns into rogue primary to a flare of arthritis.

➤ HORMONAL DISTURBANCE – Rheumatoid arthritis is greater common in women. Female hormonal elements are implicated as a causative element. Hormonal imbalance is also implicated in a flare of RA.

➤ INJURIES – Any injury can purpose a flare of RA.

➤ SMOKING – Smoking is implicated each as a causative agent in addition to a motive of flare.

➤ POLLUTION – Air and water pollutants are being postulated as a danger difficulty for flare of RA.

Many causes are despite the fact that unknown, and studies is being completed to recognize various factors which bring about flare of RA.

LAB TESTS MAY SUGGEST DISEASE FLARE OR DISEASE ACTIVITY IN RA

Rheumatoid hobby infection interest is gauged with the aid of a aggregate of signs and signs and inflammatory markers like ESR and CRP. However, ESR and CRP are not touchy or unique markers of ailment interest in RA. These markers can be raised because of more than one different factors. Many instances, those markers may be normal but the immoderate sickness hobby. Thus, it should be a aggregate of signs and signs and symptoms and signs and symptoms on the facet of correct interpretation of inflammatory markers with the useful aid of a treating scientific health practitioner that determines the disorder hobby in RA.

•A flare of RA can also result in excessive pain, disturbance, sleepless nights, absent from paintings and monetary loss.

•It shall slowly however in fact motive joint harm.

•So, it is vital to perceive the signs and symptoms (as said above) early.

MEASURES TO CONTROL FLARE

> Patients with RA have to bathtub with lukewarm water which shall lower ache and stiffness.

> Patients with RA flare should lessen/manage strain, which can be completed through meditation, yoga, challenge a calming hobby, talking to a chum or relative.

> Inadequate sleep will increase RA signs and signs and symptoms and in the long run precipitates flare. Thus, sufferers with RA

must take suitable sufficient sleep which, decreases the chance of RA flare. Adequate sleep at some point of a flare moreover enables lower RA signs and symptoms and symptoms and signs.

> There are sure food that would flare RA. However, those food are hard to emerge as privy to. Patients want to keep away from canned juices and drinks, sugary meals and processed carbohydrates. These food prompt infection inside the body and as a cease result can precipitate a flare.

Chapter 8: Emotional And Psychological Aspects In Rheumatoid Arthritis And Its Management

Rheumatoid arthritis is a commonplace disease which influences many human beings in the worldwide. RA can have an effect on any organ of the frame together with coronary coronary heart, kidneys, lung, liver, nerves, eye and so forth. If no longer treated, those sicknesses can be lethal. Rheumatologists are experts who are informed to cope with them fine.

Mental fitness consists of of emotional and mental properly being. Psychological problems along with despair, mood changes and anxiety are common in sufferers with arthritis and autoimmune diseases. A observe (Jacob et al. Depression Risk in Patients with Rheumatoid Arthritis in the United Kingdom. Rheumatol Ther 2017;4, 195–2 hundred) conducted in Britain decided that inner 5 years of RA diagnosis, about 30-35 percentage of sufferers increase melancholy. Another emotional country normally visible in sufferers of RA is tension, that is seen in 21% to 70%.

According to the research at Mayo Clinic, untreated despair and mental troubles should make it extra hard to cope with Rheumatoid arthritis. Such patients commonly have a propensity to pass pills due to melancholy. It may additionally have an effect on non-public relationships and paintings normal performance. These sufferers are greater vulnerable to repeated recurrence of immoderate ache. Thus, it is as crucial to deal with arthritis as is your intellectual health.

HOW TO ATTAIN EMOTIONAL AND PSYCHOLOGICAL WELLBEING IN PATIENTS SUFFERING FROM RHEUMATOID ARTHRITIS?

There are many distinctive aspects which need to be taken care of. A holistic method is needed for remedy of such sickness. These measures lower the dependence on capsules and act as adjunct inside the control of RA. I is probably explaining approximately all such problems underneath numerous headings as underneath -

a) How to grow to be aware of emotional health in rheumatoid arthritis

b)Managing mental elements and terrible wondering in rheumatoid arthritis

c) Stress management in rheumatoid arthritis

d)Importance of balanced existence in handling psychological and emotional aspects in sufferers of rheumatoid arthritis

e) Role of sparkling sleep, diet and exercising in managing mental and emotional elements in rheumatoid arthritis

1.IDENTIFICATION OF EMOTIONAL AND PSYCHOLOGICAL WELL BEING -

When you sense down, fear or anticipate excessively, the ones feelings can many a time restriction your capacity to look after yourself. It can also moreover limit your ability to manage your arthritis. It also can moreover affect your emotional health. Pain, intellectual fitness and disability are strongly related. Recognizing your symptoms and signs and symptoms and symptoms is the number one and maximum crucial step.

The questions beneath shall help you understand emotional and mental nicely-being -

- Are you satisfied or experience unhappy?

- Are you taking element in life or not?

- Do you feel tired even at rest?

- Do you've got got smooth sleep?

If your response is horrible, then you definately surely are emotionally and psychologically disturbed.

2.MANAGING PSYCHOLOGICAL ASPECTS AND NEGATIVE THINKING IN PATIENTS OF RHEUMATOID ARTHRITIS

Negative questioning can bring about melancholy, anxiety, fear or hopelessness.

Negative thinking might be managed thru way of following strategies –

a)VISUALIZING SOLUTION

Visualize your self that you have pop out of the undertaking you had been going to perform. This will imbibe excellent electricity in you. You may additionally need to really perform your mission with calm and ease.

b)POSITIVE SELF TALK

To defeat the terrible questioning, you need to speak to your self certainly. Think opposite of the lousy even though you get.

Example - If you get horrible thoughts that you aren't going to shop for groceries – absolutely maintain telling yourself that I may be able to purchase groceries.

c) PSYCHOLOGIST OR PSYCHIATRIST APPOINTMENT

However, in case your signs and symptoms are immoderate or no longer getting managed with the above measures inform your treating physician or ask for a referral to a psychiatrist or psychologist. In addition to the above measures, many sufferers could require medicinal capsules for management in their mental symptoms and symptoms.

3.STRESS MANAGEMENT IN RHEUMATOID ARTHRITIS

Stress is a threat component for lots illnesses like hypertension, diabetes, coronary heart sicknesses and lots of others. Stress additionally precipitates arthritis and autoimmune illnesses. It may also additionally moreover bring about fibromyalgia or continual ache syndrome.

One need to take all of the measures to lessen strain with a view to save you above said sicknesses. I will pressure upon some measures to lessen strain.

Stress buster strategies –

a)MEDITATION

Meditation is a manner that if practiced for at least 10 minutes steady with day, can help control pressure and reduce tension. Patients of fibromyalgia acting meditation each day shall advantage. Reducing stress levels will no longer simplest decrease the hazard of cardiovascular illnesses but also prevent flare of arthritis and improvement of chronic ache syndrome.

b)JACOBSON'S RELAXATION TECHNIQUE

Jacobson's relaxation approach specializes in tightening and relaxing precise muscle organizations in collection. This approach associated with the muscle businesses have to lighten up the thoughts as properly. The method includes tightening one muscle organization whilst maintaining the rest of the body comfortable, after which freeing the tension on that muscle. It permits in coping with tension and is one of the mentioned remedy options for chronic ache syndrome or fibromyalgia.

c)RELAXATION ACTIVITIES

Sitting in a park, looking T.V., films and so forth will help decrease pressure and help in controlling pressure.

d)TIME MANAGEMENT

If one manages time well, strain may lower routinely.

Some methods to control time –

•Schedule the entirety

•Give a while in your mattress/ rest

•Prioritize your artwork

e)SOCIAL SUPPORT

Family and pals are top notch guide to an character. Meeting them makes your mind and frame loosen up. Attending capabilities and occasions could make humans shed off strain.

four.BALANCED LIFE

People attention on art work and similarly paintings for that reason dropping a stability in existence. Restoring work existence stability allows lessen pressure, tension and depression. People need to prioritize lifestyles and need to cognizance on number one desires in life. To stay a balanced lifestyles, one ought to reputation on –

a)Career improvement and growth

b)Personal improvement and mastering

c)Social growth and development

d)Physical boom and improvement

A person who's living a balanced life shall lead a worrying existence.

Mild to moderate emotional and highbrow troubles are without issues controlled by using using the above measures. However, sufferers may additionally moreover moreover require psychiatrist referral or medicinal pills in early illness. Kindly inform your signs and signs and symptoms and signs and symptoms in your treating health practitioner who will manual whether or no longer medicinal pills are wanted for emotional and mental assist.

five.ROLE OF REFRESHING SLEEP, DIET AND EXERCISE IN MANAGING EMOTIONAL AND PSYCHOLOGICAL ASPECTS IN RHEUMATOID ARTHRITIS

Sleep, weight loss plan and workout play an critical feature in dealing with arthritis in addition to highbrow and emotional factors in patients of rheumatoid arthritis.

a)REFRESHING SLEEP

Studies show that as many as eighty% of humans with rheumatoid arthritis have sleeping problems. Most of the sufferers do no longer sleep nicely or don't have sparkling sleep or enjoy tired when they awaken. Patients frequently characteristic sleep troubles to ache but sleep, pain and infection flow hand in hand and it's a multi directional relationship amongst them. Those sufferers who don't get proper sleep often land up in despair or tension disorders. Sleep disturbance increases the arthritis and autoimmune ailment by way of the use of developing infection inside the frame.

Ways to normalize your sleep -

•Relaxation workout like meditation, deep breathing, Jacobson's relaxation technique

•Avoiding day time sleep

•Sleep hygiene - having a quiet sleep environment, keep away from caffeine, unique stimulants, nicotine, alcohol, immoderate fluids, or stimulating sports activities earlier than bedtime

•Cognitive behavior remedy, biofeedback remedy, paradoxical goal therapy as taught through a psychologist or psychiatrist

•Medications prescribed with the useful resource of psychiatrist or doctor

Thus it's far very critical to speak on your treating physician about sleep so that he manages your rheumatoid arthritis higher.

b)DIET

Several research have validated strong correlations amongst a healthful food plan and highbrow properly-being. Diet wealthy in smooth fruits and veggies is associated with improved happiness and higher highbrow health and nicely-being. There are many studies which show that sufferers who eat Mediterranean healthy eating plan rich in omega fatty acid, cease cease result and veggies are much much less vulnerable to anxiety and melancholy.

There are studies which show that dietary deficiencies like vitamins and minerals reason dementia and despair. Deficiencies of healthy dietweight-reduction plan B12, thiamine, niacin, eating regimen D and folic acid cause terrible mind and nerve improvement and shall cause melancholy, anxiety and emotional lability. Thus, looking after pretty a few the ones elements of weight loss plan and vitamins can help beautify emotional imbalance; lessen stress, anxiety and melancholy.

c)EXERCISE

Physical hobby and exercising can in issue save you and decorate symptoms of melancholy, anxiety, low mood and emotional imbalance. Depression and anxiety effects in will increase in inflammatory reaction. Physical hobby and workout training assist in increasing anti-inflammatory reaction and due to this manipulate despair and tension.

Chapter 9: Role Of Exercise, Joint Protection Maneuvers & Activities Of Daily Living In Patients With Rheumatoid Arthritis

Rheumatoid arthritis is a persistent disorder requiring lifelong remedy. Treatment dreams embody pain alleviation and gradual down the interest of RA to prevent deformity, incapacity and growth realistic capacity of the patient.

ROLE OF EXERCISE IN PATIENTS WITH RHEUMATOID ARTHRITIS

Most RA sufferers be troubled thru an stepped forward loss of muscle tissue which contributes to disability and worsens the terrific of existence of sufferers. In addition, RA is related to expanded morbidity and death from cardiovascular infection. It has been located that RA sufferers do an awful lot less exercising than their wholesome people. The bodily kingdom of no interest of RA sufferers is a vicious circle within the way of health and disease development.

Exercise lets in patients address chronic pain and disability with the resource of growing flexibility, persistence, type of movement (ROM), muscle & bone electricity, bone integrity, prevents cardiovascular sickness, coordination and stability. Research has installed that workout lets in to alleviate symptoms of rheumatoid arthritis. However, one should communicate to his/her medical physician earlier than beginning an exercise software program. Patients can comprise a combination of flexibility, style of movement, cardio and strengthening bodily activities.

BENEFITS OF EXERCISE IN RA INCLUDES -

✓ Protect the joint from further damages

✓ Provide pain alleviation

✓ Prevent deformity disability

✓ Increase useful capability

✓ Improve flexibility and strength

✓ Increase range of movement

✓ Improve contemporary fitness

✓ Prevent/Improves heart illnesses, diabetes and brilliant issues

✓ Improves emotional and intellectual nicely being

Which sporting activities a affected person of RA should do?

✓ Gentle bodily exercising

✓ Aerobic workout like swimming, strolling, cycling (excellent if his/her frame is healthy enough)

✓ Strengthening workout as light weight schooling

✓ Generalized stretching and range of movement sports activities

WHICH EXERCISES ARE FEASIBLE FOR ACUTE PHASE (DURING JOINT PAIN & SWELLING) IN RA

•Perform exercise at the least as quickly as an afternoon

•Gentle assisted motion via regular variety (joint Mobilisation) need to be completed at all of the joints

•Isometric "static muscle contraction" enables to maintain muscle tone without growing contamination

WHICH EXERCISES SHOULD BE DONE DURING CHRONIC PHASE (NO/MILD JOINT PAIN OR SWELLING) IN RA

✓ Light resistance bodily games want to be performed

✓ Postural / middle stability bodily activities need to be accomplished

✓ If your frame allows, swimming, on foot, cycling ought to be finished to hold cardiovascular fitness

✓ Gentle stretches for regions that become tight, which includes knees & calves need to be done

ROLE OF YOGA IN RHEUMATOID ARTHRITIS

Yoga is a exercise that includes poses, respiratory techniques and meditation. It started out in historic India and is belief as a manner to decorate bodily and intellectual health. Yoga has showed to help humans with arthritis improve many bodily symptoms like pain and stiffness, and mental troubles like stress and tension. People with various styles of arthritis who workout yoga regularly can lessen joint pain, enhance joint flexibility and characteristic, and decrease strain and tension to sell better sleep.

JOINT PROTECTION IN PATIENTS OF RHEUMATOID ARTHRITIS

In 60% of RA affected person's purposeful capability decreases within the first five years from evaluation and insideyears 50% sufferers enjoy problems in family duties.

Joint protection is a strength of will method that permits keep practical potential of joints thru changing on foot strategies of affected joints. This can be finished with the assist of high quality gadgets alongside aspect splints, changed utensils or improving the moves. Thus, converting the strolling strategies can lessen ache and pressure that is executed to the joints inside the route of day by day activities. These joint protection techniques lessen the harm & tear inside the joints and as a give up end result prevent joint harm. By modifying paintings strategies and environments, use of assistive devices (assistive generation) and inclusion of breaks within the ordinary, pain may be decreased every at relaxation and motion. Strengthening the peri articular muscular tissues and maintaining joint sort of movement through the use of exercise, moreover make contributions in a massive way to the safety or development of the affected character's useful functionality.

Joint safety techniques consist of –

1.PLANNING: Proper making plans in advance than doing a bit can decrease the try and deliver most output.

1. Do the maximum art work at that point of the day if you have minimal or no pain.

2. Try to perform a touch paintings online example- paying payments.

3. Start with more difficult obligations.

4. Break the workload and take relaxation in amongst paintings.

2.DON'T IGNORE PAIN: During exercising or even as walking in case you feel pain (extra than everyday) do now not forget approximately it. Respect pain; alternate your pastime in case you sense pain. Thus forestall sports activities if you feel which you are reaching a soreness point. Limit sports which motive ache to remaining for half of of to 1 hour submit interest. Excess ache may additionally suggest active contamination or joint damage. Do are looking for recommendation out of your doctor right now.

three.BALANCED WORK: Too plenty relaxation will boom the signs and signs of RA. Too masses art work/hobby will increase the ache and can precipitate RA flare. Thus a stability desires to be created among art work and relaxation simply so RA signs and symptoms live in remission. Patient can rest in advance than feeling worn-out. Adequate rest intervals want to be planned at some point of tough or lengthy work.

4.ADEQUATE JOINT MOTION AND MUSCLE STRENGTH: Maintaining precise sufficient joint form of movement and muscle power is of pinnacle significance for any patient of arthritis. Once style of movement and muscle energy begin to decline the frame talents decline too. Patients with RA have to accumulate complete form of movement at each joint. Patients want to moreover carry out weight training to maintain muscle strength.

5.JUDICIOUS USE OF JOINTS: To carry out responsibilities, sufferers with RA must art work with unaffected joints as an lousy lot as feasible. Use of large joints like shoulder, elbow, knee and hip makes paintings smooth and cushty for the patients. During the extreme segment activities which incorporates hiking stairs should be averted.

6.AVOID PROLONGED POSITIONS: Keeping a joint in a specific role for a long time will growth joint stiffness and for this reason joint ache. Thus, try to preserve all of the joints cellular and trade positions. Getting up out of your table at everyday periods will help save you joint and muscle stiffness.

7.WALK CAREFULLY: Rheumatoid arthritis patients have prone or osteoporotic bones. Fall poses huge chance to keep a fracture. So, those patients want to walk or do their sports activities very carefully. If the body movements nicely, stress on the joints may be averted and for that reason the danger of fall decreases. Patients ought to no longer be in a rush to do their work.

8.MAINTAINING HEALTHY BODY WEIGHT: Healthy frame weight prevents cardiovascular disease, continues rheumatoid arthritis sickness interest beneath control, and decreases the dose and amount of medicine used to deal with RA. In addition, wholesome weight decreases pressure and stress on joints and consequently prolongs the life and efficacy of joints.

9.WEAR SPLINTS/BRACE: Wearing a splint or a brace quickly to dump the stress on joints can prevent joint harm. Splints can be used to immobilize small joints just so relaxation may be given to the supportive systems.

HOW TO PROTECT HAND JOINTS

Hands and wrists are typically affected joints in sufferers of RA. Hands are the most critical structures with the useful resource of which we perform regular sports. Hand and wrist protection want to be covered. Some methods to shield hand and wrist joints are –

1. Use comfortable grip in place of a decent preserve near. Release hand grip frequently if possible.

2. Use of massive diameter pens, utensils with thick handles can reduce ache of gripping. Use adaptive equipment which includes jar openers.

3. Use the palm of your hand to open the lid of a jar. Place palm on jar lid, and use body weight to show your arm at shoulder.

4. Avoid weight relating to knuckles – it is able to harm the joints.

5. Use every fingers whenever possible.

6. Avoid extended durations of palms in a single feature. Change position often to avoid joint stiffness. Release grip often at the same time as writing.

7. Soak your hand in warmth water to relieve pain.

8. Use thick dealt with and lengthy enamel brushes, spoons and so on

nine. Large barrelled and rubber pens can be used for writing.

ACTIVITIES OF DAILY LIVING

• Walking – human beings with taking walks issues might also use walkers, stick and lots of others

•Climbing stairs – sporting foot, ankle, knee and decrease lower again assist may help some people

•Kneeling, bending, stooping – keep away from and use lengthy handles as an opportunity

•Good Grooming – use velcro and elastic in place of buttons, shoe laces and many others

•Hygiene – use excessive rest room seats, handlebars for sup- port

•Gripping – adaptive gadgets like built up door knobs and with levers and so forth

DO's

✓ DO relaxation for at least one hour within the afternoon even as you begin to enjoy fatigued

✓ DO put on nicely prepared foot put on prescribed for you (soak up surprise)

✓ DO use ice bag to reduce pain; study a heating pad or take a warm shower to lighten up muscle companies earlier than exercising

✓ DO use to be had devices that will help you with dressing, bathing, cooking, running, and awesome sports activities

✓ DO make changes, at home and paintings, for your tempo in completing obligations, to hold electricity

✓ DO check for incapacity blessings in case you are eligible or in case you couldn't artwork

✓ DO perform muscle strengthening sporting occasions as quickly as infection diminishes

DON'Ts

✓ DO NOT live in bed longer than vital

✓ DO NOT hold to place on an orthotic tool this is uncomfortable or does no longer healthy

✓ DO NOT overdo exercising. Daily exercising in small portions is best

✓ DO NOT preserve workout in case you experience pain after moderate wearing activities – record to health practitioner

✓ DO NOT workout a joint this is swollen

✓ DO NOT neglect approximately to exercising regularly whilst disorder is in remission

✓ DO NOT stay at domestic all day; in case you don't exit to paintings, be a volunteer or be part of an sports activities sports business enterprise

✓ DO NOT maintain your fears and troubles about your fitness, or feelings of disappointment or depression, to your self. Talk to circle of relatives, buddies, or your scientific medical doctor.

ROLE OF HOT AND COLD FOMENTATION IN RHEUMATOID ARTHRITIS PATIENTS

Hot and bloodless fomentation can lower pain and stiffness within the joint, for that reason supplying symptomatic remedy to the sufferers. Warming the joints before exercising and utilizing bloodless after the workout can ease the signs and symptoms and signs and symptoms and signs of joint pain and swelling.

Hot and cold fomentation has particular roles which can be as follows-

Heat treatment for rheumatoid arthritis

Heat relaxes muscle companies, reduces the pain stiffness joints and will increase blood go together with the glide and for that reason is beneficial for patients of rheumatoid arthritis. Heat treatment at the same time as mixed with sports activities will boom the style of movement of joints.

Ways to use warmth treatment –

1. Warm tub or bathe - soaking for 15 to 20 mins in a warmth tub lets in the weight-bearing muscle groups to loosen up consequently decreasing pain and stiffness. To expand the effect of a warm bathe or bath, put on warmth garments.

2. Moist heating pad

3. Soaked damp folded towels dipped in heat water (to prevent burn, continuously test the temperature earlier than the use of it).

4. Paraffin tub – Can be utilized in session with a physiotherapist.

Chapter 10: Diet Modifications And Maintaining Adequate Body Weight In Patients With Rheumatoid Arthritis

Diet performs a first-rate feature in keeping a healthful body. Unbalanced food regimen is a danger detail of many diseases like diabetes, immoderate blood strain, deranged ldl cholesterol, weight issues, coronary coronary coronary heart sicknesses, fatty liver and lots of more. Diet plays an essential role in controlling the inflammatory response this is generated in patients of arthritis. Diet plays a superb characteristic in stopping contamination flare and controlling disorder. However, there are many myths triumphing within the society about which weight-reduction plan is beneficial and that's risky. In this article I may want to located forth the scientific data approximately the beneficial and threatening food plan for patients with rheumatoid arthritis.

I might be discussing -

(I). DIETARY INTERVENTIONS USEFUL IN RHEUMATOID ARTHRITIS

(II). DIET THAT MAY INDUCE OR MAKE RHEUMATOID ARTHRITIS WORSE

(I). Dietary interventions beneficial in patients of RA –

Diets which have shown to be beneficial in arthritis are as take a look at –

a)VEGAN DIET

b)SEVEN DAYS FASTING FOLLOWED BY VEGAN DIET

c)MEDITERRANEAN DIET

d)ELIMINATION DIET

e)DIETARY FIBRE AND WHOLE GRAINS

f)FRUITS

g)SPICES

h)ESSENTIAL FATTY ACIDS

i)GREEN TEA

j)GLUTEN FREE DIET

okay)ANTI OXIDANTS

l)Nuts

a)VEGAN DIET

Intake of nice fruits and vegetables, disposing of any animal product or its with the aid of manner of-products is a vegan diet regime. Vegan weight loss plan has demonstrated to lower inflammation and due to this decrease arthritis hobby. Studies claim that the improvements in sickness interest are the result of discount in immune-reactivity to positive food antigens in the gastrointestinal tract that have been removed with the aid of adopting a vegan diet regime. Vegan food regimen additionally plays an important function in lots of different illnesses specifically patients with cancers.

b)SEVEN DAYS FASTING FOLLOWED BY VEGAN DIET

It is proved that subtotal fasting with a restrained quantity of carbohydrate and electricity collectively with nutrients and mineral supplementation and vegetable juice allows in reducing joint swelling, joint pain and irritation. Fasting period of 7-10 days with partial nutrient intake in form of vegetable broth, natural teas, garlic and decoction of potatoes, juice extracts from carrots, beets and celery. This needs to be accompanied via manner of managed every day electricity consumption followed by means of 1 year of vegan diet decreases joint ache and swelling at the side of inflammatory markers as ESR and CRP.

c)MEDITERRANEAN DIET

Mediterranean eating regimen is wealthy in anti-inflammatory and anti oxidant meals. It consists of oleic acid, omega-three fatty acids, unrefined carbohydrates, nuts, culmination, greens and plant products. Incorporating excessive portions of olive oil, cereals, end result, greens, fish, and legumes and mild quantities of red wine in diet regime decreases joint pain, swelling and will increase physical talents. Red meat, sweets and fried ingredients want to be prevented. Use of olive oil in food plan decreases the danger of developing rheumatoid arthritis. Olive oil blessings joints in addition to prevents coronary coronary heart illnesses. Mediterranean food plan has validated combined consequences. Some research have favored its feature in RA; but some studies have now not examined any decrease in contamination. However, Mediterranean eating regimen has all the anti inflammatory and anti oxidant homes and ought to advantage the patients of arthritis and autoimmune ailments.

d)ELIMINATION DIET

Many patients whinge that when ingesting sure food their arthritis symptoms and signs and signs worsened. Certain meals and its components might also additionally get worse the disorder. Thus, eliminate those meals related antigens that could in all likelihood worsen the sickness symptoms. Studies have showed that meals allergens are one of the triggers of the immune device that growth infection and because of this get worse symptoms and symptoms of arthritis.

How to discover such antigens –

1. Personal experience of meals that worsens arthritis

2. Identifying allergen antigen via pores and skin prick check

Eliminating allergen food for as a minimum eight weeks can be beneficial in controlling signs and symptoms of arthritis.

e)DIETARY FIBRE AND WHOLE GRAIN CEREALS

Some research located an inverse courting among intake of dietary fiber and inflammatory biomarkers consisting of ESR & CRP which may be signs and symptoms of inflammation in patients of rheumatoid arthritis. However, some research did no longer discover dietary fibers and complete grain cereals beneficial in reducing joint infection. Foods wealthy in whole grain and fiber are whole wheat, whole rice, oats, corn, rye, Barley, millets, Sorghum, canary seed, and wild rice. Whole grains provide rich quantities of antioxidants, phytic acid, weight loss plan E, selenium, many vitamins and minerals. These components are worried in anti inflammatory techniques and help the frame in restoring infection to regular ranges. Dietary fibers and entire grains are in any other case encouraged for their health promoting. Thus, nutritional fiber and entire grain cereals should be consumed frequently irrespective; a person is healthful or diseased.

f)FRUITS AND VEGETABLES

Bioactive components and phytochemicals, found in end result and veggies have mounted to decrease the signs of many ailments which incorporates arthritis, diabetes, bronchial asthma and coronary heart diseases. Regular intake of end result rich in phytochemicals reduces oxidative strain and infection. Fruits and flora with excessive anti oxidant and anti inflammatory residences are – avocados, dried plum, black rice, black soybean, grapefruits, banana, grapes, oranges, apples, cherries, blueberries and spinach. These end result with anti inflammatory houses help in reducing infection in sufferers of RA. Vegetables are wealthy in phytochemicals, anti oxidants and contain anti inflammatory molecules. Broccoli, spinach, advocado, cabbage, sprouts, bell peppers, carrots and mushrooms are a few vegetables that have above cited houses.

g)SPICES

Ginger, turmeric and cinnamon bark have proved to be useful as anti-inflammatory sellers every in rats and human research. Turmeric has an energetic compound known as curcumin which reduces joint pain and swelling. However, they need to be enthusiastic about heat materials as warmness milk a good way to increase the absorption of those substances and are absorbed in big portions to motive anti-inflammatory movement. Spices have additionally been utilized in conventional treatment for treating many ailments. Spices are mills of bad strength as they growth metabolic rate. Ginger and chillies are beneficial on this regard.

h)ESSENTIAL FATTY ACIDS

Omega three fatty acid has a excessive anti-inflammatory assets. They have showed to lower joint pain and swelling in numerous types of arthritis which embody rheumatoid arthritis. Fish oils, flaxseed oil, walnut oil, mustard oil, olive oil, soybean oil, canola oil and corn oil are some of the oils wealthy in omega 3 fatty acid and characteristic anti inflammatory homes.

i)GREEN TEA

Green tea has substances that have mounted function in prevention and treatment of cardiovascular sickness. It blocks inflammatory pathways and as a result possesses anti inflammatory houses. It is placed to decrease joint swelling to some extent.

j)GLUTEN FREE DIET

Gluten is a substance in fantastic food like wheat which reasons allergy and induces irritation within the body. Scientific facts concerning gluten loose weight loss plan and its function in arthritis is inconclusive in the intervening time.

okay)ANTI OXIDANTS

Role of antioxidants like food plan C, vitamins A, zinc and selenium in arthritis is dubious. Some studies favour reaction at the same time as others do not.

* NUTS

Nuts as almonds and walnuts have anti-inflammatory homes and due to this reduce irritation in joints. Anti-inflammatory healthy dietweight-reduction plan now not most effective decreases frame's infection but moreover will increase electricity levels within the frame. Anti-inflammatory eating regimen may also help the affected person to shed pounds.

(II). Diet that could result in or make arthritis worse

Following listing of food that are dangerous in arthritis

a)SWEETENED SUGAR SODA

b)FRIED AND PROCESSED FOOD

c)SUGAR AND REFINED CARBOHYDRATE

d)SMOKING

e)HIGH SALT AND PRESERVATIVES

a)SUGAR SWEETENED SODA

Sweetened soda has been associated with an extended hazard of rheumatoid arthritis. When in assessment to <1 sugar-sweetened soda in step with month, consumption of ≥1 sugar-sweetened soda in line with day has sixty three% prolonged chance of growing rheumatoid arthritis. Thus, sugar sweetened soda and merchandise containing the identical want to be prevented.

b)FRIED AND PROCESSED FOOD

Decreasing fried and processed meals shall reduce contamination and assist restore the frame's herbal defence.

c)SUGARS AND REFINED CARBOHYDRATE

High quantities of sugar in food plan can motive irritation in the frame and get worse arthritis symptoms and symptoms. Thus, the equal desires to be avoided in the diet.

d)SMOKING

Smoking not most effective will increase the risk of coronary heart assaults and cancers, it furthermore will increase the risk of improvement of rheumatoid arthritis. People with arthritis who smoke are prone to lung involvement. Smoking is mainly prohibited in sufferers with arthritis.

e)HIGH SALT AND PRESERVATIVE RICH DIET

Some studies suggest that healthy eating plan rich in salt and preservatives get worse inflammation and therefore worsen arthritis.

ANTI-INFLAMMATORY DIET SHOULD CONTAIN –

1. 25 gram of fiber consistent with day

2. 2 servings of fruits and seven servings of vegetables (1 serving = equates to half of of a cup of fruit or cooked greens or one cup of raw leafy veggies)

3. Whole grain cereals

four. Avoid alcohol

5. EAT FOUR SERVINGS OF ALLIUMS AND CRUCIFERS WEEKLY (Alliums consist of garlic, scallions, onions and leeks, on the identical time as crucifers talk to veggies which

includes broccoli, cabbage, cauliflower, mustard greens and Brussels sprouts)

6. Consume omega three wealthy food

7. Cook with herbs and spices

8. Avoid processed meals and sugars

9. Avoid saturated fats and trans fat

10.Use unsaturated fats and oils

CONCLUSION

In nutshell, one should maintain on with the anti inflammatory weight loss plan - need to encompass greater end result and vegetables, keep away from fried and sugary meals. Alcohol wants to be averted, smoking is honestly prohibited. One want to hold healthful weight and do everyday exercising. There is not any constant diet plan this is tested for RA patients. What works for one person may not art work for distinctive. Hit, trial and errors assist one determine which meals one want to put off from diet. The function of weight loss program has its boundaries. It can't update the function of medication. It has installed benefits but as an accessory to medicinal capsules. Definitely, it could decrease the quantity and dose of medicine with the beneficial useful resource of reducing irritation and consequently reducing sickness interest. However, earlier than starting a contemporary healthy dietweight-reduction plan or food a affected individual need to consult his/her health practitioner as nutritional modifications can cause horrific interplay with drug treatments.

MAINTAINING ADEQUATE BODY WEIGHT

Weight control is an important a part of anybody's existence. People who hold the right weight for his or her age and pinnacle basically experience a healthful life. They are less inclined for immoderate ailments like diabetes, coronary coronary heart assaults and many others. Similarly, weight management plays a completely vital function on top of factors of RA patients.

IMPORTANCE OF WEIGHT LOSS IN RA

• Reduce strain for your joints therefore lessen pain

• Reduce contamination in frame and joints

• Reduce Disease Activity in RA

• Reduces hazard of RA flare

• Slows Cartilage Degeneration in joints

• Decreases dose/shape of drug treatments

• Reduces chance of comorbidities which include diabetes, coronary coronary heart illness.

Chapter 11: Quality Of Life In Rheumatoid Arthritis & Ways To Improve It

Quality of life as defined by the usage of the World Health Organization (WHO) method, "man or woman's perception in their role in lifestyles in phrases of way of life and systems wherein they stay, in terms of their dreams, expectations, requirements and issues".

Quality of lifestyles includes - physical health, mental united states of america, diploma of independence, social relationships, personal ideals and their relationships.

Rheumatoid arthritis impacts multidimensional elements of existence. RA impacts the bodily health due to joint pain and deformities. Patients frequently aren't able to perform everyday responsibilities. RA additionally affects emotional and highbrow factors of existence. Changes in self-notion when it comes to painful stimuli, decreased useful ability, and labour and social inadequacy also can bring about emotional and intellectual troubles.

As RA impacts a couple of domain names of lifestyles therefore tremendous of lifestyles questionnaires in RA embody all the ones domains. Quality of existence questionnaires in RA encompass - the bodily dimensions (pain and deterioration of bodily functioning), the highbrow dimension (anxiety and despair), the cognitive length (interest and reminiscence) and the social size (conceitedness and interpersonal relationships).

STRATEGIES TO IMPROVE QUALITY OF LIFE IN RA PATIENTS

1. Disease recognition – It has been visible in research that the patients who receive the illness and begin dwelling with it have better remarkable of life then people who don't be given the disorder as a part of themselves. Thus, accepting ailment early and starting remedy prevents joint damage and because of this prevents deterioration of extremely good of lifestyles.

2. Early remedy – Early diagnosis and treatment prevents joint deformities, much less chance of growing melancholy and anxiety. Patients are capable of do all of the sports activities associated with personal and expert lifestyles.

3. Achieving low disorder interest – Low disease interest or disease beneath control is associated with better brilliant of lifestyles then patients with slight to excessive disease hobby.

four. Empowering sufferers of RA - Empowerment facilitates the sufferers assume considerably to have the possibility to make self enough and knowledgeable selections as a manner to get what they want, address ordinary existence and decorate excellent of lifestyles. The empowered sufferers used their statistics of having had a protracted-time period scenario for several years, and had a perception in their very very own capability to govern one-of-a-kind conditions, and a manner to reset dreams and expectations. Empowering a affected character of RA permits enhance the great of existence of the sufferers.

five. Social help - Accessibility of diverse social relationships and participation with circle of relatives, buddies and co-people improves high-quality of lifestyles of sufferers with RA

6. Continuing professional - Continuing the expert paintings and preserving ones engaged improves the best of lifestyles of sufferers.

7. Sleep – Disturbed or insufficient sleep is associated with negative extraordinary of life in assessment to sufferers with a normal sleep pattern.

8. Anxiety & despair – Patients with RA who boom tension and melancholy lead bad extraordinary of lifestyles. However, as soon as each these problems are underneath manipulate the satisfactory of lifestyles of a RA affected character improves.

9. Emergency health finances – RA sufferers may moreover broaden health emergencies

subsequently of their existence. Thus, a few amount of cash should be saved apart as an emergency fund.

DISEASE ACCEPTANCE

Acceptance is considered as adjustment, model or negotiation with continual ache. It turns into very essential to simply accept the ailment because of the fact recognition is step one to control disorder/continual ache.

Sequences in accepting a persistent disease consist of - turning into privy to the hassle and receiving a analysis; acknowledging the chronicity of the pain and the following losses; and putting in a new manner of dwelling.

Studies have tested that illness reputation performs a super role in sufferers' bodily, social and emotional functioning. It has been visible in numerous studies that the patients who come to phrases with ache record greater best clinical results, more self assurance of their coping capability, higher each day uptime, a good deal much less melancholy and lots a lot much less ache. They respond better to remedy and stay a better quality of life.

Earlier the recognition, the better it's miles for the patients with RA. Accepting the illness early and starting normal remedy prevents joint damage and therefore prevents surgical treatment or headaches of rheumatoid arthritis.

It has been visible that the higher the amount of sickness beauty, the more self sufficient and active the affected character is. The patients who have everyday their situation commonly take delivery of the want of remedy and additionally don't forget their scientific personnel. By now not accepting the illness, one dangers making subjects a good buy worse for oneself.

Chapter 12: Real Life Scenarios Of Rheumatoid Arthritis Patients

There are many actual lifestyles case summaries of patients which inform us the significance of early analysis and ordinary treatment in rheumatoid arthritis. I would be sharing such stories truely so human beings are advocated and do no longer lose preference.

Case1

•Patient A – age – forty two yrs, starting of RA signs and symptoms for the purpose that 1 three hundred and sixty five days

•On ordinary remedy and examine up for 7 years

•Currently – no joint damage or any organ involvement, dwelling a wholesome regular life, quality on 2 pills constant with day, going to place of business

Lesson learnt – Early evaluation and ordinary treatment help hold joints, danger of involvement of main organs of the body like coronary coronary heart, thoughts, lung, and so on decreases, sufferers require tons less tablets to manipulate sickness and affected character is able to carry out all his household and expert work independently.

Case 2

•Patient B —32 years age, beginning of RA symptoms and symptoms considering that 1 yr

•Was doing nicely on drugs, left treatment as she desired medicinal drug unfastened illness manipulate

•Visited after 7 years – moderate to mild deformities and joint damage

•Had lung involvement

•Requires multiple capsules which includes biologicals and oxygen remedy for lung involvement

Lesson learnt – Patient was identified early and turn out to be doing properly on drug treatments. Patient left remedy superior joint harm and lung involvement. Patient required organic remedy collectively with multiple drugs and oxygen in a while.

Case three

•Patient C- forty years age, Disease length – 10 years – strange treatment

•Severe joint damage – need to require knee joint alternative

•Developed stroke or paralysis due RA

Lesson learnt – weird treatment ends in joint damage and will increase the danger of paralysis due to swelling/inflammation in blood vessels because of RA

Case 4

•Case of RA age 50 years – 15 years illness length – did no longer take proper remedy - knee modified – doing properly on drug treatments – publish surgical treatment – doing all her sports activities, going to workplace

•Living a healthy lifestyles with drugs

Lesson learnt – Irregular remedy results in out of manage illness which could damage joints. Once joints are critically damaged surgical treatment may be required. Patients can lead a healthy unbiased lifestyles submit knee opportunity with drug remedies for RA by myself.

Case 5

•Case of RA – age – 28 years, ailment signs and symptoms and symptoms while you bear in mind that 5 years, affected character on regular treatment due to the reality that 5 years taking oral drugs. However, infection however not controlled with oral drug remedies, sufferers require herbal treatment. Patient has the equal opinion for the same, given herbal remedy.

•Patient's sickness is virtually underneath control. Better reaction to oral drug remedies and organic remedy stopped.

Lesson learnt – Biological remedy even as used at proper time can manipulate the illness and consequently prevent joint harm.

Case 6

•35 twelve months male – RA for the cause that 5 years

•Initially wrist and palms worried – have become better with drug remedies – left remedy – pain swelling restarted – took pain killers – after 6 months visited medical institution all over again as disorder have come to be excessive and unfold to all joints – began drug remedies – became higher after 6 months – self medicating – got here after 1 twelve months with lung involvement and joints requiring replacements and biological treatment. Patient moreover superior diabetes.

Lesson learnt – Irregular treatment ends in out of manage illness that can damage joints and lungs. Such sufferers can also moreover require better remedy as natural. RA if out of control posses a huge risk of growing diabetes, coronary coronary heart attacks and so on.

Case 7

•RA considering the truth that 10 years – uncommon and now not on time treatment – knee joints damaged – changed (3.Five lacs), lung concerned – required common hospitalization because of lung infections or breathing difficulties, require luxurious drug treatments for treatment

Lesson learnt – Irregular and delayed remedy motives out of control disease which possesses danger of joint damage and recurrent hospitalisations because of stepped forward danger of infections due to out of manage RA.

Chapter 13: Importance Of Regular Visits To A Doctor

Many instances a affected person thinks why to visit a medical doctor while he/she is doing tremendous. But, it's miles very critical to go to a health practitioner frequently as he advises because of multiple motives –

1. Doctors want to check whether or not or now not the illness is really underneath manage or is contemporary.

2. Every medical doctor has a plan for each of his/her sufferers to reduce the quantity of medicine whilst a affected man or woman is doing well on a particular set of drugs.

3. During each visit a scientific physician needs to check whether or not his/her affected character is growing aspect results or headaches (involvement of coronary coronary heart, lung, kidney, nerves, eyes etc) of ailment. If that trouble is detected early it will be reversed surely.

four. During every visit a health practitioner checks whether or not or not his/her affected man or woman develops any thing consequences of medicine or no longer.

5. The medical doctor exams whether or now not the affected man or woman is developing any comorbidity like diabetes, excessive blood strain, weight problems, heart troubles and so on.

6. Time to time, a scientific physician advises the life-style modifications for his/her sufferers.

Chapter 14: Medicines To Treat Rheumatoid Arthritis Patients

With improvement in medical technological know-how, there may be extremely good development in the control of rheumatoid arthritis. Gold and penicillamine which had been as soon as taken into consideration gold elegant for the remedy for RA have turn out to be topics of the past. Newer and more secure capsules are available to treat patients of RA. Newer drug treatments are extra efficacious and feature plenty lots much less facet outcomes even though charge of those drug remedies stays a trouble in most of the locations.

An vital detail is – one medication may fit well for one affected individual and might not paintings for each other the equal way. Sometimes it can take a twelve months orfor the medical doctor to find out which remedy awesome fits a selected patient. Give your clinical medical doctor time to discover what works brilliant for you.

Medicines used to deal with RA are -

•Anti inflammatory drug treatments – Non steroidal anti inflammatory pills - NSAIDS (pain killers), Steroids

• Traditional DMARDs (Disease enhancing anti rheumatic drugs)- Methotrexate, Leflunomide, hydroxychloroquine, Sulfasalazine

•Biological DMARDs - TNF blockers (infliximab, eternacept, golimumab, adalimumab), Tocilizumab, Rituximab, Abatacept

•Oral organic - Tofacitinib, Baricitinib

•Iguratimod and Immunosuppressant pills - Mycophenolate mofetil, Azathioprine, Cyclophosphamide, Tacrolimus

1.Anti inflammatory drugs -

This beauty of drug remedies encompass of medicine which is probably beneficial for the sufferers in lively or flare up of RA. This beauty of medication are used till the time the primary DMARDs begin appearing. The drug treatments on this elegance are slowly tapered off and can be used once more while ailment flares up. These drugs are for use accurately via the treating medical doctor.

2.Traditional DMARDs (Disease improving anti rheumatic capsules)-

This elegance of medicine used to cope with RA includes – methotrexate, sulfasalazine, leflunomide and hydroxychloroquine. These drug remedies due to the fact the decision shows are disease enhancing this is they forestall disease development of RA. They no longer only save you ailment development however furthermore prevent RA patients from infections with the aid of the use of using controlling the disorder. They moreover save you RA patients from getting more articular manifestations like coronary coronary coronary heart assault, stroke and masses of others. These drug remedies are gradual to act and take three-6 months to reap complete effect.

3.Biological DMARDs

Biological DMARDs is a category of drugs which may be cutting-edge-day drug remedies with excessive efficacy to govern RA. These tablets typically act speedy and control sickness in a way that they prevent disorder development. These drug treatments are normally indicated whilst traditional DMARDs fail to govern the sickness hobby. These medicines are a piece expensive injectable drug treatments which can be given with the aid of intravenous course or subcutaneous path. The drug remedies on this group include of –

a) TNF Blockers – Adalimumab and its biosimilars, Infliximab and its biosimilars, Golimumab, eternacept and its biosimilars

b)IL-6 inhibitor – Tocilizumab

c)IL-1 inhibitor – Anakinra

d)Fusion molecule – Abatacept

e)B mobile depletion - Rituximab

4.JAK KINASE INHIBITORS

These are quite greater moderen lessons of oral tablets which have dramatically changed the manipulate of RA. These drug treatments are as a substitute efficacious medicines to deal with RA.

5.IGURATIMOD

This is a new magnificence of medication used to cope with patients of rheumatoid arthritis. This remedy is but now not popular for use in all global places.

6.IMMUNOSUPPRESSANT DRUGS

Immunosuppressant drug remedies in RA play a exquisite role while RA has unfold beyond joints. These are beneficial while RA has involved lungs, eyes, kidneys, mind and nerves and lots of others. Medicines in this class embody mycophenolate mofetil, cyclosporine, cyclophosphamide, tacrolimus and azathioprine.

WHEN AND HOW MUCH RESPONSE TO EXPECT IN RA

Response to remedy in rheumatoid arthritis depends on multiple elements – most important of that's how early the treatment has been initiated after beginning of disorder signs and symptoms.

Other factors rely on the diploma of joint harm, the bodily practical popularity of the affected person, mental fitness, and the presence of comorbid infection which includes cardiovascular illness, contamination, and B cellular lymphomas.

Treatment reaction in state-of-the-art is gradual in patients of RA. It is anticipated that almost all of patients ought to take 3-6 months to get the symptoms to normalise. It is to be considered that 30-forty percent of patients obtained't reply to the ordinary (traditional/conventional DMARDs) tablets used to cope with RA. In the ones sufferers better remedy as herbal DMARDs or JAK kinase inhibitors need to be introduced.

Moreover, an essential aspect for the affected individual to have a look at isn't all sufferers reply to the same drug remedies. Also, no longer all patients respond in addition to all drug remedies. Doctors want to find out that is the first-rate cocktail of medicine with a view to be the handiest for a affected person. Sometimes to find out the equal, it could take months to a one year or .

It has been tested that a 33% discount of radiographic/sickness development in sufferers of RA who became treated earlier than 2 years disease length in assessment with those dealt with later. These benefits have been sustained as an entire lot as 5 years.

Long time period very last consequences (10 year) of dealt with patients with early arthritis (an entire lot much much less than 2 twelve months length) modified into assessed in multiple research. Ninety four percent of these treated early and frequently had been able to do all their features through themselves at 10 years.

Response is sustained within the ones sufferers who're on ordinary remedy in place of taking intermittent drug remedies.

SIDE EFFECTS OF MEDICINES TO TREAT RHEUMATOID ARTHRITIS

Rheumatoid arthritis is a controllable illness. Medicines are an important element to manipulate sickness hobby of RA. If the illness stays uncontrolled it shall damage the joints and purpose disability and deformity. Not simplest joints, out of control sickness can also moreover damage essential organs of the body like coronary coronary heart, thoughts, lungs, nerves, eyes and so forth. These aspect consequences of sickness will rise up in almost a hundred percent of the sufferers of RA if the disease stays untreated.

Medicines used to deal with RA are critical to manipulate disease interest. As said – now not a few element is 100% secure on this universe. Neither the food we consume (food can reason contamination and many first rate ailments), nor the drug treatments. There is a danger of aircraft getting crashed whilst we excursion. Similarly, the medicines are not a hundred percent safe. However, those drug treatments to address RA were studied in animals and people and the problem impact of those capsules is widely recognized. These aspect effects don't arise in every man or woman. Serious component consequences of those drug treatments are uncommon and occur in 1 in masses or lacs of sufferers. There are techniques to screen those issue outcomes of medicine used to address RA. By normal monitoring, we can find out the ones facet consequences early and can be outcomes reversed.

I will be discussing some side consequences of medication used to cope with RA along side measures via which we are able to avoid detail outcomes of drug treatments.

Medicines

Side Effects

Watch Out For

Monitoring/ Precautions

NSAIDs

Gastrointestinal ulceration and bleeding, renal damage and so forth

Blood in stool, dyspepsia, nausea or vomiting, susceptible factor,

dizziness, belly

ache, edema, weight

gain, shortness of

breath

Liver function assessments (LFT), kidney feature assessments (KFT) and urinalysis inner three months - repeat the ones studies every 6 to 365 days if low risk or each three monthly if immoderate threat (to be determined via manner of health practitioner)

Corticosteroid

Hypertension,

Hyperglycemia, cataract, weight advantage,

Osteoporosis, infections, gastric ulcers and plenty of others

Symptoms of not unusual urination, expanded thirst, edema,

seen changes, weight

advantage, nausea, vomiting, complications,

broken bones or bone

pain

Vaccinations as in keeping with your clinical physician, 3 monthly test up for sugar, weight manipulate, regular exercising, every 12 months eye test up, blood stress monitoring

Methotrexate

Nausea, vomiting, Bone marrow suppression, Increased liver enzymes,

hepatic fibrosis,

cirrhosis, alopecia,

stomatitis, rash, infections and so on

 Shortness of breath, nausea or vomiting, lymph node

swelling, coughing,

oral ulcers, diarrhea, hair fall,

jaundice

 Vaccinations as in line with your scientific medical doctor, blood assessments as Complete blood count number range range (CBC), LFT, KFT initially monthly for 3 months then each three month-to-month

Leflunomide

 Increased liver enzymes ,

gastrointestinal

misery, bone marrow suppression, alopecia, infections and so forth

 Nausea or vomiting,

gastritis, diarrhea, hair

loss, weight loss, oral ulcers, free stools, jaundice

Vaccinations as in step with your scientific scientific physician, blood exams as CBC, LFT, KFT first of all month-to-month for 3 months then every three month-to-month

Sulfasalazine

Bone marrow suppression,

Rash, stomach pain, headache and so on

Abdomen ache, headache, photosensitivity, rash,

nausea or vomiting

Blood checks as CBC, LFT, KFT to begin with monthly for 3 months then each three monthly

Hydroxychloroquine

Dark skin,

rash, itching, diarrhea, now not frequently deposition in eye and so on

Visual changes

along with a lower

in night time or peripheral

vision, rash, diarrhea

Yearly eye test up through an ophthalmologist

Etanercept,

Adalimumab,

Anakinra

Infliximab,

Rituximab,

Abatacept

Local injection-web internet site on-line

reactions, infections,

Immune reactions and so on

Symptoms of contamination like fever, prolonged cough, parasthesia, postinfusion reactions etc

Vaccinations and blood checks as normal together with your medical doctor

Tofacitinib, baricitinib

Herpes zoster, Herpes simplex, Gastroenteritis, Urinary tract infections, thrombocytosis, nausea and so forth

Fever, pores and skin rash, belly ache, vomiting and so forth

Vaccinations and blood assessments as steady together along with your health practitioner

Mycophenolate mofetil

•Stomach pain, nausea, vomiting, unfastened stool, constipation,

•bleeding gums,

•itching, numbness, prickling sensations, low blood counts, multiplied chance of infections and so forth

 Watch out for multiplied frequency of stools, stomach pain, loose stool, vomiting, hair fall, and masses of others

Chapter 15: Blueprint To A Pain Free Life Amongst Patients With Rheumatoid Arthritis

Rheumatoid arthritis is a persistent disorder requiring lifelong remedy in most of the times. As referred to in previous chapters it's far combined attempt from each medical health practitioner & affected person that can exchange the life of RA patient to a ache loose life. I shall be discussing about the steps a RA affected man or woman want to have a look at to stay a ache free existence.

STEPS WHICH A PATIENT SUFFERING FROM RHEUMATOID ARTHRITIS MUST FOLLOW TO LIVE A PAIN FREE LIFE -

1. First and maximum essential problem which a affected person of RA have to apprehend is that he/she suffers from a sickness known as rheumatoid arthritis. This illness is incurable just like maximum distinct sicknesses (diabetes, multiplied blood pressure, thyroid issues, kidney, coronary heart, lung diseases and so forth). However,

incurable does now not mean that there may be no remedy available for the identical. There are suitable and superior medicines which might be now resultseasily available that would manage the disorder and save you complications. Thus, sickness recognition is the maximum & most critical step.

2. Second step closer to a pain unfastened life is to visit a representative for RA treatment. Rheumatologists are professionals who are properly professional to cope with RA.

3. It has been seen that the sufferers who start treatment early are capable of live painless or life with slight ache compared to sufferers who do away with their remedy or have advanced deformities or complications. So, starting early is the important thing to living a pain free existence.

4. Further, trusting your medical physician is the following step. Your doctor shall prescribe you medicines depending on the extent of your ailment. Sometimes natural treatment can be required to control the sickness.

He/she can also additionally order assessments on a normal c programming language to look for facet effects of illness or drug remedies.

five. Following proper way of existence modifications play an essential position in controlling the illness. Once a affected character adjusts his/her lifestyles consequently, then simplest he/she can be able to gain ache loose lifestyles.

Lifestyle changes which a patient of RA need to comply with are – ordinary exercise, maintaining properly enough frame weight, consuming a balanced anti-inflammatory weight loss plan, taking good enough nicely timed sleep, following joint protection techniques and sports of every day dwelling.

6. Patients tormented by rheumatoid arthritis are at progressed chance of growing psychiatric manifestations as melancholy and anxiety. These elements need to be managed well with self motivation strategies as described in this ebook. If self motivation

strategies aren't adequate to govern psychiatric manifestations then patients want to are trying to find advice from a systematic medical doctor for the identical.

7. Controlling co morbid infection as thyroid illnesses, diabetes, coronary coronary heart illnesses and so forth assist reduce ache inside the body. Adequately controlling co morbid infection plays an crucial feature in dwelling a pain unfastened existence.

8. Regular examine up is each different fundamental difficulty of remedy of RA. It has been seen that those sufferers who observe their medical doctor often are at lots a good deal less threat of growing thing outcomes of disorder or the drug treatments. The disease in those patients receives controlled early and calls for fewer drug remedies.

In brief it need to be a everyday sustained try from every scientific doctor and affected individual which permits one to stay a pain free lifestyles amongst patients with rheumatoid arthritis.

Chapter 16: Background To Rheumatoid Arthritis

Pathology; Signs and Symptoms

Rheumatoid arthritis exerts its amazing effect at the joints lined with synovium, the tissue responsible for keeping vitamins and lubrication of the joint, inflicting contamination and the signs of joint ache and swelling. The distribution of synovial joints tormented by RA is likewise function of the ailment, and it typically impacts the small joints of the palms and the ft, and typically every components further in a symmetrical distribution. However, any synovial joint of the body may be affected particularly as soon as this competitive sickness is installed.

The impact of the infection effects in a massive increase in blood go together with the glide to the joint (giving off heat and occasionally redness), proliferation of the synovial membrane with an boom in synovial fluid (swelling), and pain (because of stretching of ache receptors inside the gentle tissues spherical, and the bone on each element, of the joint). This consequences in rapid lack of muscle round an affected joint, and this, on the aspect of pain and swelling outcomes in lack of joint feature. In the absence of suppression of the synovial membrane contamination there can be growing damage to the joint, due to the release of protein degrading enzymes from inflammatory and special cells. Increasing damage to the joint is also because of conversion of factors of the synovial membrane into an inflammatory tissue known as pannus that could invade the bone

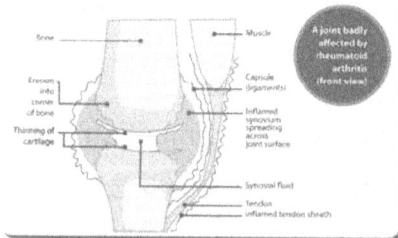

Figure 1. A joint affected by rheumatoid arthritis

and cartilage at the margins of the joint, and furthermore the connecting bone surfaces end up eroded (Figure 1).

The degree of contemporary damage is related to the depth and duration of the irritation. Damage to joints effects in revolutionary deformity, incapacity and handicap. Other structures with synovial linings, which incorporates tendon sheaths, can be affected as properly, and infection of these can result in tendon rupture.

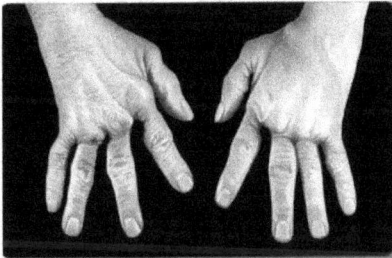

Figure 2 Hand of person affected by rheumatoid arthritis showing joint swelling and deformed positions of fingers and thumb

Suppression of infection within the early levels of the sickness can result in large improvements in lengthy-time period results for joints and special components of the musculoskeletal gadget. However, even when the infection is managed, the effects of swelling due to the construct-up of fluid in the capsule of the joint are irreversible. The tablet remains stretched and consequently cannot preserve the joint in position making the joint with the ensuing uncommon or deformed positions which is probably a exquisite clinical characteristic of set up RA (Figure 2 and Figure three).

Another characteristic of RA is the rheumatoid nodule or "necrotizing granuloma" sometimes visible over bony prominences of the hand, or regions that preserve repeated mechanical strain. The nodule has a vital place of fibrinoid necrosis

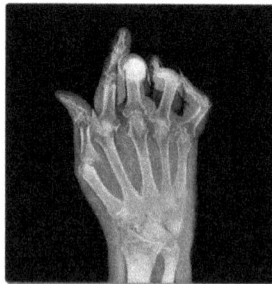

Figure 3. X-ray of hand of person with rheumatoid arthritis

that can be fissured and which corresponds to the fibrin-rich necrotic cloth positioned in and round an affected synovial vicinity. Nodules are related to a tremendous RF titer and excessive erosive arthritis.

A Systemic Disease

Rheumatoid arthritis is in truth a systemic disorder. In everybody with RA the discharge of huge concentrations of proteins that power the inflammatory methods, in conjunction with tumor necrosis issue-α, (TNFα), bring about signs of profound fatigue, ongoing influenza-like signs, or even fever, sweats and weight reduction. Furthermore, special frame organ systems can be affected by the inflammatory technique, with dryness of the eyes and mouth (Sjögren's syndrome), and nodules (difficult lumps specifically over extensor surfaces similar to the backs of elbows) and this can have an effect on as much as a 3rd of people with RA.

Inflammation of the joints additionally may be existence-threatening whilst it affects the neck, inflicting in all likelihood volatile articulations among the bones, and inflammatory pannus and absence of mobility. The combination of bone deformity and swollen inflammatory tissue can motive pressure at the spinal twine, leading to ischemia and big neurological effects affecting all four limbs, bowel and bladder characteristic, or the respiratory muscle businesses and centers inside the mind stem that manipulate respiratory, with capability fatal results. Although the ones lifestyles-threatening inflammatory results of RA are uncommon, and are probably turning into rarer due to superior early assessment, scientific management and remedy, to be alerted to them makes one privy to the potential excessive effects of this illness.

More excessive systemic outcomes additionally can be manifested, which embody fibrosis in the lungs, infection affecting the lining of the coronary coronary heart and lungs (pleural and pericardial effusions), or vasculitis. Vasculitis outcomes in inflammation of the inner lining of the blood vessels and might result in likely devastating outcomes for whichever organ is furnished thru the affected blood vessels. Examples of vasculitis are scleritis of the attention, a painful and probable sight threatening vasculitis, and peripheral neuropathy, wherein nerves are irreversibly damaged most important to weak spot or sensory abnormalities.

Moreover, it has end up more and more obvious that the persevering with infection and loss of mobility have to have awesome surprising results with severa unique excessive diseases being not unusual in people with RA. Heart conditions collectively with ischemic coronary coronary heart sickness and cardiac failure have been installed to be extra not unusual in RA. Indeed, atherosclerosis is driven in issue via ongoing irritation, simply so the human beings with the maximum active RA have the pleasant hazard of coronary coronary coronary heart illness. Osteoporosis is likewise not unusual in human beings with RA, because of a combination of reduced mobility and contamination. Osteoporosis is likewise an unfavourable impact of a few RA remedies, for instance the glucocorticoids, despite the fact that those tablets will be inclined now fine to be prescribed for quick-time period remedy of contamination thereby lessening their unfavourable consequences.

People with RA are greater susceptible to infections than the general population. This is in detail due to abnormalities inside the immune device, but is likewise resulting from immunosuppressant results of some RA treatment, for instance the glucocorticoids, however furthermore the new natural response modifiers (biologics). Indeed, human beings taking biologics should be immunised in opposition to commonplace contamination diseases earlier than starting off treatment.

Preclinical Rheumatoid Arthritis

The initial cause for RA is unknown. There is evidence to indicate abnormalities in components of the immune device that cause the frame growing everyday immune and inflammatory reactions, specially in joints.

These modifications can also moreover precede the symptomatic onset of RA through a few years. ACPAs and RF gift numerous years earlier than ailment onset suggests a slow machine main to the development of RA.Nine Soluble immunological markers also are superior closer to the onset of signs and symptoms indicating activation of the immune device. Understanding of preclinical RA may additionally moreover assist those at risk, assist the statistics of the etiology of the illness and can assist improvement inside the path of improvement treatments and possibly a therapy. Genetic markers for RA can be stated in the subsequent monetary break.

Methods of Classification

The class standards superior in 1987 through the American College of Rheumatology (ACR)10 have been the identical vintage for RA class for decades, and were primarily based on an assessment of past due-stage features, along with erosive joint sickness and staying electricity of signs (Table 1). The standards have advocated clinical workout, and had been utilized in countrywide scientific pointers as lots as very currently.Eleven,12 However these necessities were no longer designed for scientific exercising, neither were they to be diagnostic. They had been formulated as a difficult and speedy of criteria to standardise the elegance of RA in scientific research. The certainly one of a kind important interest is

Table 1. Summary of 1987 classification criteria for rheumatoid arthritis (Source: Arnett, Edworthy et al. 1988)

that the requirements do now not embody any evaluation of the early degrees of RA, i.E., early synovitis which has turn out to be an increasing number of critical to the evaluation of RA and the upgrades in remedy, specifically taking off therapy as early as possible with DMARDs. Indeed, for that reason some international locations have not used the 1987 standards of their pointers and alternatively use a clinical assessment, considering this to be more vital than assessing whether or not or not a type requirements are glad.

Revised Classification Criteria (2010)

The 1987 necessities have now been surprisingly revised to cope with early disease. These new requirements had been produced together with the European League Against Rheumatism (EULAR) as part of an global collaboration.Thirteen This new type tool makes a speciality of capabilities at earlier tiers of infection which is probably associated with persistent and/or erosive disorder. This brings the requirements into line with the critical want for in advance assessment and early powerful disorder-suppressing treatment to prevent or restriction the prevalence of the unwanted sequelae that comprised the actual standards.

The new necessities redefine RA, reflecting the authors' collective desire that inside the destiny, RA will not be characterised with the useful useful resource of erosive joint disorder and staying energy of signs and symptoms, even though those tendencies will maintain to define established or longstanding untreated disease.

In the contemporary requirements set, category as "actual RA" is primarily based totally on the confirmed presence of synovitis in as a minimum 1 joint, absence of an opportunity diagnosis that better explains the synovitis, and success of an entire rating of 6 or greater (of a probable 10) from the man or woman ratings in four domains: amount and location of worried joints (rating range 0–5), serologic abnormality (rating range 0–3), accelerated acute-section response (rating variety 0–1), and symptom period (2 ranges; variety 0–1) (Table 2).

The authors13 aspect out that the category scheme is designed to give a standardized approach to identifying the subset of folks that present with in any other case unexplained peripheral joint inflammatory arthritis, for whom chance of symptom endurance or structural harm is sufficient to be considered for intervention with DMARDs. They pressure that the requirements are supposed handiest for eligible patients in whom the presence of apparent clinical synovitis in as a minimum one joint is precious, and the requirements want to no longer be implemented to sufferers with arthralgia or to regular subjects. Hence, the elegance scheme is the today's proposed paradigm for the entity "rheumatoid arthritis", however importantly, not standards for "early" RA. They nation that if there has been an intervention that come to be each infinitely powerful and safe and can be supplied without fee and no soreness, then there might be no requirement for this form of subset to be diagnosed, as each affected character with inflammatory arthritis is probably dealt with. Given that such an intervention does no longer exist, the look for suitable class rules is justified, and also will be beneficial in guiding medical analysis.

As with all hastily developing regions of drugs, a impediment of any new requirements is that they're based on cutting-edge know-how, which relying upon inclinations can swiftly turn out to be previous. The authors commentary that genetic, proteomic, serologic, or imaging biomarkers that offer a better basis for chance stratification and identification of immoderate-chance groups may additionally moreover emerge, and this can always bring about a exchange or amendment of the 2010 requirements. An example is the brand new biomarker, ACPA to be able to be noted later in the chapter on chance factors.

Again the ones criteria are labelled "elegance requirements" in choice to "diagnostic requirements." As stated above, the reason is to provide a standardized approach for discriminating, from a populace of human beings offering with undifferentiated synovitis, the subgroup with the pleasant opportunity of chronic or erosive RA, who may be enrolled into medical trials and distinct research thru the use of uniform necessities, and those who may also therefore advantage from DMARD intervention.

The authors nation that the necessities do no longer dispose of the onus on character physicians, especially in the face of unusual and wider indicates, to accumulate a diagnostic opinion that might be at variance from the challenge acquired using the requirements. Nonetheless, they recognize that the contemporary-day requirements will

likely moreover be used as a diagnostic aid.

Notes:

* The requirements are aimed toward elegance of newly presenting patients. In addition, patients with erosive ailment wellknown of RA with a records well matched with previous fulfillment of the 2010 standards need to be categorised as having RA. Patients with longstanding illness, inclusive of these whose illness is inactive (without or with remedy) who, primarily based on retrospectively to be had information, have previously fulfilled the 2010 requirements should be categorized as having RA.

† Differential diagnoses range amongst patients with unique indicates, but may embody situations which incorporates systemic lupus erythematosus (SLE), psoriatic arthritis, and gout. If it's far doubtful about the applicable differential diagnoses to don't forget, an expert rheumatologist have to be consulted.

‡ Although patients with a rating of <6/10 are not classifiable as having RA, their popularity can be reassessed and the requirements is probably fulfilled cumulatively over the years.

§ Joint involvement refers to any swollen or easy joint on examination, which may be confirmed through imaging evidence of synovitis. Distal interphalangeal joints, first carpometacarpal joints, and primary metatarsophalangeal joints are excluded from assessment. Categories of joint distribution are labeled consistent with the region and quantity of concerned joints, with placement into the satisfactory class viable primarily based absolutely on the pattern of joint involvement.

¶ "Large joints" refers to shoulders, elbows, hips, knees, and ankles.

"Small joints" refers to the metacarpophalangeal joints, proximal interphalangeal joints, second thru fifth metatarsophalangeal joints, thumb interphalangeal joints, and wrists.

** In this class, as a minimum 1 of the worried joints want to be a small joint; the alternative joints can include any aggregate of massive and further small joints, in addition to precise joints not specifically indexed a few vicinity else (e.G., temporomandibular, acromioclavicular, sternoclavicular, and masses of others.).

†† Negative refers to IU values which might be less than or same to the pinnacle restriction of everyday (ULN) for the laboratory and assay; low-excessive excellent refers to IU values which may be higher than the ULN however ≤3 times the ULN for the laboratory and assay; immoderate-terrific refers to IU values that are >three times the ULN for the laboratory and assay. Where RF facts is only available as excellent or bad, a fantastic cease result ought to be scored as low-powerful for RF.

‡‡ Normal/uncommon is determined thru neighborhood laboratory requirements.

§§ Duration of signs refers to affected character self-record of the length of symptoms and signs and symptoms or signs and symptoms and signs and symptoms and signs of synovitis (e.G., pain, swelling, tenderness) of joints which can be clinically worried on the time of evaluation, regardless of treatment reputation.

Diagnostic Tests

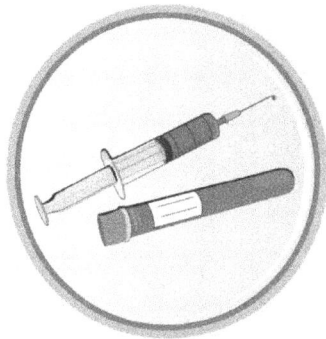

No single take a look at can supply a specific analysis of RA in the early ranges of the scenario. Doctors need to attain at a analysis based totally totally on symptoms and symptoms and signs and symptoms, a bodily examination and the outcomes of x rays, scans and blood assessments (see area).

Because RA may want to have an effect on numerous body systems it's far critical the affected character describes all symptoms.

Chapter 17: Risk Factors And The Search For Possible Causes

Risk Factors for Rheumatoid Arthritis

Both non-modifiable and modifiable chance elements make a contribution to the improvement of RA. Non modifiable threat elements encompass age (RA much more likely with increasing age; top of onset 30-fifty five years), gender (much more likely in ladies than men) and genetic factors, and modifiable hazard elements encompass oral contraceptives, pregnancy, weight loss program, infection, career and smoking. The unique mechanisms wherein the ones hazard factors result in clinical illness live doubtful, and a few are certainly showed as risk elements and some are despite the fact that considered functionality elements.Five

Genetic Factors

Much of this improvement in information the pathogenesis of RA has involved elucidating the complex interactions a number of the innate and adaptive immune systems, which have vital roles inside the onset and perpetuation of synovitis in RA, for example the presence of autoantibodies, RF and ACPAs, in asymptomatic people up to ten years preceding to the arrival of scientific disorder.Five RA predominately develops in genetically predisposed people, but, for the reason that RA is a heterogeneous sickness there may be however a awesome deal variation in predisposing elements and clinical presentation. The genes inherited from mother and father can also have an effect on the opportunity of growing RA, but genetic factors on my own do no longer reason RA. A character with an equal dual who has RA, does no longer suggest they will too amplify the disease for which the hazard is 1 in five. The genetic contribution to RA debts for approximately 60% of the variant in liability to disorder.14 The most crucial genetic danger predisposing a person to RA is the splendor II vicinity (especially genes encoding human leukocyte antigen-D related [HLA-DR] molecules) of the crucial histocompatibility complex (MHC) locus, and make up approximately 13% of the overall genetic variance.15

Proven risk factors for RA embody genetic affects on the characteristic of the innate and adaptive immune systems, smoking, ACPAs, and RFs; functionality threat factors encompass epigenetic manage of gene expression, the microbiome and different environmental factors, Toll-like receptors, cytokines, and Fc receptors.Five However, the correct mechanisms in which those risk elements purpose clinical disorder stay uncertain. Arend and Firestein america that it is possible that, combined with activation of the innate immune machine, a subset of ACPAs initiates the disease in the cartilage or synovium after binding to endogenous citrullinated proteins. Subsequent engagement of Fc receptors and supplement activation could result in secondary infection in the synovium with induction of a perpetuating cycle of continual synovitis.

Smoking

Smoking is the maximum fantastic and characterized environmental risk detail for RA and damage is incurred over a few years in a genetically predisposed host.5,sixteen It is proven that the mixture of SE alleles and smoking is related to RA susceptibility regardless of ACPA or RF repute, but that the combination shows stronger results in ACPA–awesome/RF-satisfactory patients with RA than in ACPA–negative/RF-awful sufferers with RA. The shared epitope–smoking interactions have been found in ACPA–powerful and RF-remarkable RA. Although smoking consequences in citrullination of lung proteins, the mechanisms whereby cigarette smoke or extraordinary noxious stimuli set off those inflammatory activities are but to be defined.

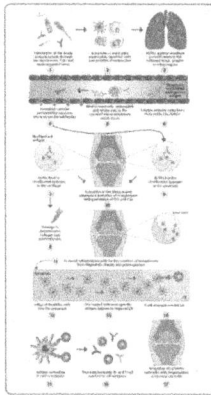

Figure 4. Proposed mechanism of initiation of RA (Source: Arend and Firestein 2012)

A further paper thru De Hair et al. (2012) describes the number one potential observe showing that smoking and obese increase the hazard of development of arthritis in a cohort of autoantibody-high-quality individuals at threat for developing RA. These effects show the significance of life style elements in improvement of RA and ought to be notably evaluated in destiny scientific studies aimed in the direction of ailment prevention.

The determine shows that a couple of preclinical immune and inflammatory activities finally exceed a threshold after which clinical sickness is initiated: 1) Repeated episodes of stimulation of the innate immune device, consequences in 2) activation of myeloid cells, and likely chondrocytes. Three) Local infection in mucosal-blanketed organs ends in ACPA production. Four) ACPAs bind to exogenous or changed endogenous antigens to shape circulating immune complexes that 5) have interaction with myeloid cells within the synovial microvasculature and tissue. 6) Increased vascular permeability effects, with diffusion of autoantibodies into the joint. 7) ACPAs bind to specific citrullinated epitopes in the cartilage 8) predominant to damage to cartilage additives. Nine) ACPAs can also bind to citrullinated epitopes within the synovium. 10) In every web sites, the classical and alternative pathways of complement are activated. Eleven) Synovium infection is added approximately with infiltration of macrophages main to similarly citrullination, enzymatic and oxidative harm to structural proteins and advent of neoepitopes. 12) DCs loaded with joint-specific antigens are gift within the synovium and procedure the altered self-peptides, after which thirteen) migrate to community LNs in which 14) T-mobile activation to start with occurs. 15) Epitope spreading follows over time with the development of sixteen) actual autoimmunity. 17) Chronic synovitis ensues through activation of cytokine networks. Key: ACPA, anti-citrullinated protein antibody; DCs, dendritic cells; LN, lymph node; RA, rheumatoid arthritis; TLR, toll-like receptor.

Assessing the Causes

Rheumatoid arthritis often seems after a latent period of a few years therefore the reasons of the disease cannot be determined with the useful resource of way of reading the signs and signs and symptoms, e.G., infected joints, by myself and lots statistics gained from epidemiological research is contradictory or indistinct.18 Of the modifiable chance factors with possible or in all likelihood links to RA, best cigarette smoking has been examined epidemiologically.18 Obviously this hyperlink presents proof for the significance of lifestyle adjustments and health education throughout the problems of smoking. Moreover, reading the immunological profiles of patients with RA who smoke and/or have been uncovered to cigarette smoke may furthermore assist provide information across the reasons of this disease.

It is likewise vital to recollect the occurrence and occurrence of RA geographically spherical the region. In a scientific evaluation of studies 1988 to 2005 inclusive reporting the incidence and occurrence of RA in person populations sixteen to 20 years and over (RA necessities based mostly on 1987 ACR Criteria) a splendid difference turn out to be discovered in incidence among northern European and American countries and growing countries.19 South European global locations had a decrease median prevalence than North American and north European global locations, however of the latter there has been evidence of reducing occurrence of RA in Finland and america. However, the as an alternative small quantity of research eligible for inclusion in this have a take a look at (28 in all; nine occurrence research, 17 prevalence research and a couple of prevalence and incidence studies), and the lack of occurrence research for the growing worldwide locations presently limits the scope for understanding the epidemiology of RA worldwide.

Rheumatoid Arthritis inside the History of Medicine

(Source: www.News-clinical.Internet/fitness/Rheumatoid-Arthritis-History.Aspx)

The first statistics of RA date lower returned to 4500 BC.

A textual content dated 123 AD describes signs and symptoms and signs and signs and symptoms very much like RA.

In 1800 the French health practitioner Dr Augustin Jacob Landré-Beauvais (1772-1840) primarily based mostly on the Salpêtrière Hospital in Paris describes instances common of RA providing first recognized description of the sickness.20

In 1859 British rheumatologist Dr Alfred Baring Garrod names the illness "rheumatoid arthritis…an inflammatory contamination of the joints, no longer in assessment to rheumatism in some of its characters, but differing materially from it in its pathology".21

However, ancient epidemiological evidence can also offer beneficial records about the genetic basis of RA as evaluated via Mobley (2004).22 Mobley's observations got here from analyzing the literature on the epidemiology of deaths because of tuberculosis (TB) from 1780 to 1900 and decided it positioned a setting immediately-line correlation to the epidemiology of RA nowadays (Figure 5). In 1886, the TB lack of lifestyles charge for Native Americans become approximately 9.Zero%, the satisfactory charge ever recorded for any population inside the international, and local Americans currently have the high-quality expenses of RA worldwide, with a incidence of 5–7%.23,24 In evaluation the TB loss of life fee in England in the course of this era became 1.2% in 1780, at the identical time as in North America, the peak loss of life rate reached 1.6% in 1800, on the equal time as in recent times those populations have RA expenses between zero.Five% and 1.Five%.25,26 In Asia costs of RA are low (<0.Three%) and from to be had opinions it might appear that expenses of TB within the 19th century had been also low. The fee of RA in rural Africa has been tested to be a exceptional deal less than 0.1%, and no times of TB are stated for the 19th century. The reality that the epidemiology of modern-day day RA is strikingly just like the epidemiology of TB a hundred–two hundred years in the past, suggests the possibility that genetic factors that superior survival in TB epidemics at the moment are influencing susceptibility to RA. Recent advances within the assessment of genetic polymorphisms associated with ailment have identified numerous genes related to RA susceptibility that encode proteins involved inside the immune response to mycobacterium TB infection, which incorporates TNFα, NRAMP1, PARP-1, HLA-DRB1, and PADI4. These consequences advocate that RA, and probable wonderful autoimmune ailments, are cutting-edge day manifestations of the genetic selective stress exerted via TB epidemics of the cutting-edge past.

Figure five. A correlation among present day-day RA incidence and TB loss of life costs in the current beyond. Death fees in 1900 for Native Americans due to TB have been obtained from the Fort Qu'Appelle location of Ontario, Canada. RA expenses for Native Americans are available for the Pima Indians (5.Three%) and the Chippewa Indians (6.Eight%). (Source: Mobley, 2004)22.

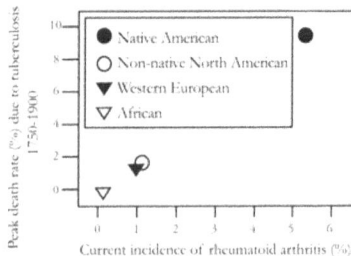

- --

Conventional Treatments for Rheumatoid Arthritis

Treatment with artificial DMARDs has big barriers including partial efficacy and horrible tolerability.2 However, combination regimens, which consist of humans with the modern-day natural often concerning weekly manipulate of the artificial DMARD, MTX due to the fact the anchor drug, were used an increasing number of to triumph over the regulations of DMARD monotherapy.27

Analgesics

Painkillers reduce pain in place of infection and are used to control the signs and symptoms and symptoms of RA. The most normally prescribed painkiller is paracetamol. Codeine is each one of a kind painkiller this is on occasion prescribed as a blended treatment with paracetamol (known as co-

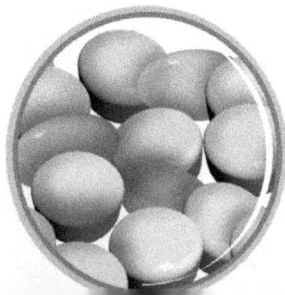

codamol).

Non-Steroidal Anti-Inflammatory Drugs (NSAIDs)

Non-steroidal anti inflammatory pills (NSAIDs) are typically used along distinctive RA capsules, to help manipulate ache, infection, and swelling related to RA; NSAIDs do now not gradual RA development.

Non-selective NSAIDs (e.G., diclofenac, naproxen, ibuprofen) act via blocking off the results of the two cyclo-oxygenase (COX) enzymes, known as COX-1 and COX-2, that stimulate the manufacturing of prostaglandins, a number of that are involved in inflicting ache and infection at net websites of damage or harm in the body. Thus the impact of the NSAIDs is to reduce the manufacturing of prostaglandins and thereby reduce pain and contamination.

Chapter 18: Glucocorticoids

Glucocorticoids (e.G., prednisone, methylprednisolone) do now not alter the direction of the sickness inside the equal manner that DMARDs or biologics do, but can be used to govern RA symptoms and signs and signs in the short-term due to the fact their impact in lowering infection is commonly rapid. For instance, glucocorticoids can be supplied as quick-term treatment for managing surprising flares in human beings with modern-day onset or installation sickness to rapidly lower contamination, as an example at the identical time as looking in advance to extraordinary pills like DMARDs to take effect.30 Glucocorticoids can be administered orally, intravenously, or can be injected right away right into a joint, as a result permit a number of alternatives for treating signs and symptoms.

It is usually recommended that in humans with established RA, glucocorticoid remedy should best be persisted whilst the prolonged-time period headaches of glucocorticoid treatment had been truely cited with the affected person, and all exceptional remedy options (which includes organic tablets) had been provided.

Glucocorticoid use is likewise restricted through the element effects they could reason, which incorporates weight benefit, muscle weak spot, excessive blood pressure, improved blood sugar, osteoporosis, temper disturbances, prolonged vulnerability to infections, and neighborhood atrophy of the pores and skin on the internet page of steroid injections, facial flushing and interference with the menstrual cycle. Doses of steroids are stored as little as possible to lower the risk of component-effects. It occasionally endorsed that calcium and nutrients D or bisphosphonates are taken concomitantly to off-set thinning of the bones.

Synthetic Disease-Modifying Antirheumatic Drugs (DMARDs)

DMARDs act with the aid of manner of treating the underlying contamination rather than the symptoms. Pain, swelling and stiffness are reduced over a period of weeks or months with the aid of slowing down the contamination and its consequences on joints. DMARDs no longer exceptional help control signs and signs and signs and symptoms, they can also decrease joint damage and stave off destiny headaches. Synthetic or conventional DMARDs encompass gold injections; hydroxychloroquine (HCQ); MTX; and sulfasalazine.

Although regularly effective, DMARDs have been restricted in treatment durability over the long term because of component outcomes and declining efficacy. However, as greater has been learnt about RA inside the previous few years, DMARDs had been delivered at earlier stages of disorder that permits you to gradual or prevent radiographic illness progression before irreversible joint harm, paintings disability, useful decline and different terrible consequences are seen.31 Furthermore, mixture regimens, which encompass people with the contemporary herbal regularly concerning weekly MTX due to the fact the anchor drug, were used increasingly more to overcome the policies of DMARD monotherapy.

The synthetic DMARDs encompass MTX, HCQ, sulfasalazine, and leflunomide. These DMARDs produce symptomatic development and slowing of radiographic development however have giant boundaries and terrible tolerability as prolonged-time period treatment.32,33 The dominant DMARD, MTX has emerged because the mainstay of treatment for RA mainly with the advent of low-dose weekly regimens (7.Five-15 mg weekly, titrated to a most of 25 mg consistent with week, and administered orally or through subcutaneous injections), and is the anchor compound in most mixture treatments.2,34 MTX is an antimetabolite that inhibits dihydrofolate reductase, an enzyme required for DNA synthesis. MTX has verified better reaction charges and progressed lengthy-term adherence in evaluation to specific synthetic DMARDs. Side consequences of MTX may be minimized with careful monitoring and the addition of folic or folinic acid.

Several combinations of artificial DMARDs were shown to be more effective than monotherapy, probable because of the truth the improved efficacy comes from simultaneous outcomes on special inflammatory pathways involved in the pathogenesis of RA. Effective combos consist of sulfasalazine, MTX, and HCQ, and leflunomide to MTX despite the fact that the latter become taken into consideration to require close to monitoring as it grow to be related to higher costs of adverse sports activities.35,36 Increased efficacy of anti-TNF sellers with concomitant MTX has been demonstrated in several randomized trials, and simply maximum of the approved anti-TNF stores are indicated in combination with MTX. There have no longer been many research evaluating TNF inhibitors with other synthetic DMARDs, but a few advocate similar hazard/benefit, for instance leflunomide in combination with a TNF inhibitor as seen with MTX plus TNF inhibitor.37 Furthermore, a 2 year scientific trial of early aggressive RA verified that triple DMARD therapy had similar efficacy to MTX in mixture with the TNF inhibitor, etanercept.38

Biologics or Biological-Response Modifiers

Developments inside the expertise of the pathogenesis of RA and the arrival of biologic restoration tactics with the functionality to particularly targeted on unmarried additives within the inflammatory cascade have considerably advanced the manage of RA in scientific exercise.39

Until 1998 (the date while the primary biologic, etanercept, turn out to be criminal for treatment of RA), artificial DMARDs, along side MTX, had been the principle trendy remedy for RA. With the advent of the natural DMARDs or biologics came a bypass inside the path of an early and competitive technique to

RA treatment. The new dealers have been overcoming a number of the restrictions of the artificial DMARDs with a extra rapid onset, superior and sustained efficacy, and functionality to inhibit the development of joint damage.

The biologics are commonly properly tolerated in terms of not unusual factor consequences, but human beings taking biologics are at advanced threat of contamination, which embody TB and persistent viral infections, and patients embarking on a course of biologics are screened rigorously and should undergo vaccination for infectious disorder. However, TB can be extra not unusual amongst people who've RA than it is inside the preferred population, and that hazard seems to be increased thru remedy with any immunosuppressive medicinal drug, now not without a doubt the ones biologics.Forty The monetary rate of biologics is also substantially better in comparison to artificial DMARDs, but, this need to be balanced in the direction verified to be an powerful treatment for RA.2 Two kinds of TNF inhibitor are to be had: a soluble TNF receptor (e.G., etanercept), and monoclonal antibodies to TNF (e.G., infliximab, adalimumab, golimumab, and certolizumab). The first of these biologics had been inhibitors of TNFα and interleukin (IL)-1, targeted on CD20 B cells or interfering with T cellular activation through blocking off CD80/86:CD28 signalling. However, it was determined that approximately 70% of patients though did now not accumulate remission and about 29–fifty four% did no longer show considerable improvement with TNFα antagonists. The improvement of remedies focused on in addition down the

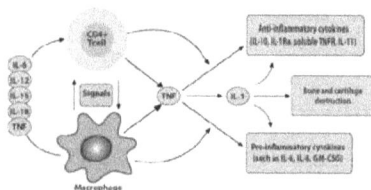

Figure 6. The cytokine network in rheumatoid arthritis (Source: Feldmann 2002)⁹

cytokine cascade, such has IL-6 has helped decorate the ones results.

TNF Inhibitors

Etanercept (Enbrel®)

Etanercept (Enbrel®; artificial with the resource of Amgen, CA, USA), have end up the number one TNF inhibitor accepted via way of the FDA for treatment of RA in 1998 (Table 3).

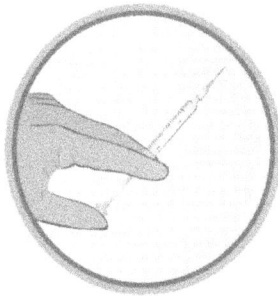

Etanercept is a recombinant fusion protein fabricated from TNF receptor linked to the Fc a part of human immunoglobulin (IgG1); it binds to TNFα and TNFβ and forestalls their interplay with cellular ground TNF receptors.[2]

The clinical efficacy of etanercept in RA emerge as set up in a important look at thru Weinblatt et al. (1999).Forty one that confirmed that etanercept and MTX provided extensively more scientific benefit than MTX by myself. Like all TNF inhibitors the efficacy of etanercept is prolonged in combination with MTX.FortyWeinblatt et al. (2011)forty 3 have moreover said effects of prolonged-time period etanercept remedy, and characteristic proven that advantages are maintained past 10 years of remedy in each early and longstanding RA patients. They advise that etanercept is properly tolerated and effective as an extended-term, non-prevent remedy for the remedy of RA, with a excellent hazard/gain ratio.

Etanercept appears to be the least immunogenic TNF inhibitor. All TNF inhibitors product labels have a black location caution for extreme infections, however the superiority of TB and probable extraordinary infections may be less with etanercept than with anti-TNF antibodies which incorporates infliximab.2 This may be because of the truth it's far a receptor and does now not bring about apoptosis in cells with TNF on their ground. Moreover, this could deliver an motive of why etanercept has minimal gain in a few off-label rheumatic illnesses along with vasculitis and uveitis. Because of its mainly quick 1/2-life (about 2.Eighty three days), immunomodulatory outcomes are extra speedy dissipated on the same time as etanercept is withheld all through intercurrent infection.

Infliximab (Remicade®)

Infliximab (Remicade®; synthetic thru Centocor [Johnson & Johnson, NJ, USA]), is a chimeric monoclonal anti-TNFα antibody composed of a human IgG1 and a variable region of a murine anti TNF antibody.

Infliximab grow to be first frequent in 1998 for Crohn's Disease and fistulising Crohn's Disease, but a 12 months later changed into conventional for the remedy of RA in mixture with MTX in sufferers with an insufficient response to MTX. Clinical and radiographic advantage of infliximab in sufferers with insufficient reaction to MTX were proven within the ATTRACT trial,forty four,forty five and in MTX-naïve patients inside the ASPIRE trial of early-onset RA.Forty six Ongoing art work through the same corporation has endured to illustrate decrease disorder development and higher rates of remission with infliximab plus MTX compared with MTX on my own.Forty seven

Infliximab has the benefit of exceptional dosing flexibility (three–10mg/kg doses by means of way of IV infusion at zero, 2, and 6 weeks, then every four–8 weeks).2 However, the IV device calls for an infusion middle management and is related to infusion reactions, that is a functionality downside in evaluation to for example, subcutaneously administered etanercept. Unlike etanercept despite the fact that, infliximab has efficacy for nice off-label indicators in conjunction with vasculitis, uveitis, and sarcoidosis, however there may be extra multiplied hazard of infections consisting of TB. Etanercept moreover has an prolonged elimination 1/2-lifestyles of about 8–eleven.6 days.

Adalimumab (Humira®)

Adalimumab (Humira®; artificial with the useful resource of Abbott, IL, USA), is a completely human monoclonal antibody (mAb) in opposition to TNFα and come to be first authorized for the remedy of RA in 2002. Its absolutely human gather offers the capability gain of reduced immunogenicity in contrast to infliximab.2

Adalimumab has a fast onset of motion and sustained efficacy (the elimination 1/2 of of-life is about 14 days), retards improvement of structural joint damage, improves characteristic, and is typically properly tolerated. Adalimumab has been showed to be clinically and radiographically effective in RA with responses visible as early as 1 week after initiation of remedy, however determined better charges of mild or slight injection site reactions and sure intense infections, together with TB, in addition to uncommon instances of non-skin cancers and important demyelinating infection.Forty eight,40 nine However, a Cochrane evaluation of six research with 2380 sufferers handled with adalimumab confirmed its efficacy, and brought into attention it safe inside the remedy of RA as monotherapy and in aggregate with MTX.50 It may additionally moreover have the gain of a 2-weekly subcutaneous dosing habitual and a completely human construct, however adalimumab nevertheless outcomes in human antihuman antibody formation, in particular if MTX is not co-administered.2

Golimumab (Simponi®)

Golimumab (Simponi®; artificial with the useful resource of Centocor [Johnson & Johnson, NJ, USA]), end up the fourth TNF inhibitor to be common for RA (FDA 2009). It is a completely humanized anti-TNF agent with an prolonged median 1/2-life starting from 7 to twenty days. It is administered monthly as a 50 mg subcutaneous injection, and this dosing schedule is its chief gain over the primary generation TNF inhibitors.1

The safety and efficacy of golimumab were evaluated to start with in three section III trials. The GO BEFORE take a look at in which golimumab changed into administered as first-line remedy of early-onset RA previous to MTX did no longer meet its number one endpoint of ACR50 response at 24 weeks, however the co number one endpoint of inhibition of radiographic improvement at 52 weeks changed into met.Fifty one,fiftyIn the GO FORWARD take a look at in which sufferers with energetic RA received golimumab and MTX, efficacy changed into sustained from 24 through fifty two weeks.Fifty three Likewise, GO-AFTER confirmed efficacy at the same time as golimumab plus MTX turned into administered to sufferers who had previously acquired anti TNF treatment.Fifty four

Certolizumab Pegol (Cimzia®)

Certolizumab pegol (CZP) (Cimzia®; artificial thru UCB [Smyrna, GA, USA]), is the 5th TNF inhibitor for RA to be authorised (USA 2009);

CZP changed into first accepted inside the USA in 2008 for the remedy of Crohn's illness.

Certolizumab pegol is a completely unique pegylated TNF alpha inhibitor (TNFi) treatment.Fifty five It is precise in form and mechanism of movement in comparison with the sooner TNF inhibitors because it consists of a polyethylene glycol (PEG) moiety, and lacks the regular fragment (Fc) of immunoglobulin; therefore it does no longer activate supplement. As well as showing clinical efficacy, there can be evidence to signify that CZP has specific inclinations, which incorporates decreased transfer during the placenta and reduced frequency of injection net web page reactions.Fifty 5

In Phase three scientific trials of slight to immoderate, active Crohn's illness, CZP became associated with drastically more reaction fees in contrast with placebo at weeks 6 and 26 after commencement of treatment.Fifty six In patients who replied to the 6-week induction, CZP administered as a month-to-month subcutaneous injection have become powerful in retaining CD response and remission. A latest review considers CZP beneficial in sufferers with slight to excessive illness.Fifty seven

Three phase III trials, the RA prevention of

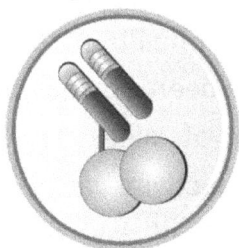

Figure 7. Simulated model of the novel pegylated TNF alpha inhibitor certolizumab pegol (Source: Melmed et al. 2008)[a]

structural harm (RAPID) 1 and a couple of studies59,60 and efficacy and protection of CZP four weekly dosage in RA (FAST4WARD) have a observe,sixty one mounted early and sustained clinical efficacy in sufferers with inadequate reaction to MTX or one among a type traditional DMARDs. An open label extension of the RAPID I test stated that scientific and radiographic gain modified into sustained after 2 years.Sixty ,sixty three,sixty four An up to date protection profile from the ones 3 trials did not display screen any new safety issues and showed CZP is just like other TNF inhibitors especially across the chance of outstanding infections.Sixty five In summary, CZP treatment substantially advanced affected character-counseled very last results measures, providing top notch reductions in ache and fatigue and upgrades in physical function as early as Week 1 of treatment; enhancements in health-associated terrific of existence have been obvious on the number one evaluation at Week 12. CZP treatment advanced productivity at work, drastically reducing the type of days of left out artwork similarly to the form of days with reduced productiveness (Figure 8), and additionally extended productivity within the domestic and improved participation in circle of relatives, social and enjoyment activities. CZP became typically nicely tolerated while used each as monotherapy or brought to MTX; most negative occasions were moderate or moderate. Taken together, the consequences of those trials recommend that CZP is an effective new desire for the treatment of RA.Sixty six,67,68

Results are verified at baseline and study stop. (A) Work days neglected (absenteeism) due to arthritis consistent with month. (B) Days with paintings productivity decreased via 550% (presenteeism) because of arthritis in step with month. (C) RA interference with artwork productivity consistent with month (0–10 scale, zero = no interference, 10 = whole interference). The assessment populace in RAPID 1 and a couple of trials became the purpose-to-deal with population (employed patients first-class). *P ≤zero.05 vs placebo plus MTX. Analyses were accomplished the use of a non-parametric bootstrap t-test and the final statement carried in advance approach.

Other Biologics

Anakinra (Kineret®)

Anakinra, (Kineret®; synthetic with the useful resource of Amgen, CA, USA), is a recombinant human IL-1 receptor antagonist protein accepted for use in RA in 2001. IL-1 blockade showed large inflammatory gain in preclinical research, but scientific revel in has observed out anakinra to be a pretty willing biologic in RA with best modest ACR responses.38,sixty nine,70 Because of the significantly low efficacy, each day dosing, and common pores and pores and skin reactions, anakinra has no longer been a main RA biologic. The mixture of anakinra and etanercept modified into associated with prolonged infections without superior efficacy.Seventy one Consequently, coadministration of anakinra and a few other biologic agent is not advocated, and stays indicated for slight to immoderate RA in adults who've failed one or extra DMARDs.

Chapter 19 : Abatacept (Orencia®)

Abatacept (Orencia®; synthetic through Bristol-Myers Squibb, NY, USA) is familiar to be used in adults with moderate to severe RA and insufficient reaction to at least one or more DMARDs. It is not used as a primary-line biologic but essentially used after failure of various biologic dealers. It is the primary immunotherapy directed in opposition to T-cell costimulation. T-mobile activation is important to the initiation and renovation of RA.2 Multiple antigens can cause the inflammatory method in a genetically willing host. Maximal T-cell responses normally require costimulation, and blockade of the costimulatory signal changed into the idea of development for abatacept. Abatacept (CTLA4-Ig) is a chimeric fusion protein composed of IgG1 Fc and extracellular vicinity of CTLA4. It blocks complete T-mobile activation by way of way of using inhibiting the CD28:CD80/CD86 co-stimulation.

Several registration trials have established the efficacy of abatacept: abatacept in inadequate response to MTX (AIM),seventyabatacept trial in the remedy of anti-TNF insufficient responders (ATTAIN),seventy 3 abatacept researched in RA patients with an insufficient anti-TNF response to validate effectiveness (ARRIVE),seventy four abatacept or infliximab in place of placebo, the trial for tolerability, efficacy and protection in treating RA (ATTEST),75 abatacept look at of safety in use with extraordinary RA treatment plans (ASSURE),76 and abatacept have a take a look at to gauge remission and joint damage progression in MTX naïve sufferers with ERA (AGREE).Seventy seven

Recent lengthy-time period open label extensions of AIM and ATTAIN trials tested sustained scientific efficacy at five years and 4 years, respectively.Seventy eight,79 However, it has a slow onset to maximum efficacy, it certainly is at three months. Its safety profile changed into similar to other biologic shops, but the combination of abatacept with each other biologic agent changed into related to an multiplied hazard of first-rate issue consequences.

Abatacept is now additionally accredited for subcutaneous administration. Subcutaneous abatacept did not elicit immunogenicity associated with lack of protection or efficacy, each without or with MTX,80 and established comparable efficacy rather than adalimumab with comparable kinetics of response and inhibition of radiographic development at 1 yr, and the protection became generally comparable aside from appreciably greater nearby injection net website online online reactions than with adalimumab.Eighty one

Rituximab (Rituxan®)

Rituximab (Rituxan®; manufactured through Genentech, CA, USA/Biogen Idec, MA, USA) is the primary of severa biologic dealers to intention B cells, which play a important function in the pathogenesis of RA. It is a chimericm antibody in the route of CD20, it is expressed on the floor of all mature B cells however no longer on plasma or stem cells.

It come to be prison for the treatment of RA in 2006 at the idea of its scientific efficacy in sufferers with lively RA refractory to MTX or TNF inhibitors,80 ,eighty three and its useful effect on structural damage.Eighty four The IMAGE trial additionally stated clinical and radiographic benefit in MTX naïve sufferers.Eighty five,86 Rituximab is not presently used as a primary-line biologic however more regularly than not carried out in TNF inhibitor failure. The principal retreatment ordinary remains uncertain because the duration of medical gain varies drastically among exceptional patients, and no surrogate marker of treatment impact has been recognized. Several modern research verified that fixed retreatment time desk also can purpose tighter control of sickness interest however can also be associated with increased component outcomes.87

The safety profile of rituximab is typically similar to awesome biologics, and a metanalysis of records from 3194 patients handled with rituximab with 11962 affected character-years of publicity stated that rituximab modified into well tolerated with none new safety concerns.88 A few times of patients on rituximab growing innovative multifocal leukoencephalopathy have been noted,89,ninety and the product label now consists of this warning. However, facts from a rustic large populace-based completely cohort have a look at in Sweden propose that patients with RA may furthermore have an improved fee of PML compared with the general populace.91

Tocilizumab (Actemra®)

Tocilizumab (Actemra®; synthetic through the use of Chugai, IL, USA/Hoffman-LaRoche, CA, USA), is a anti-IL-6 receptor humanised monoclonal antibody. IL-6 is a pleiotropic cytokine involved in B- and T-cell activation, induction of acute section reactants, and stimulation of hematopoietic precursor cellular differentiation, and is overexpressed in synovial fluid, and may contribute to joint destruction via its effect on osteoclast function. It represents a present day remedy preference in patients with mild to excessive active RA who've both spoke back inadequately or are illiberal to preceding treatment with one or more DMARDs or TNF antagonists.

In scientific studies tocilizumab come to be well tolerated and efficacious in alleviating the signs and symptoms of RA, further to inhibiting radiological development.92,903,ninety four,ninety five The effects of these studies brought about the approval of tocilizumab by the use of the European Medicines Agency (EMA) in January 2009 and by using the usage of the FDA in January 2010. It is the 9th and most cutting-edge biologic for RA. Recent prolonged-term look at-up statistics from the ones medical trials suggested developing clinical efficacy over time at some point of three.Five years of check up.Ninety six

The specific capabilities of tocilizumab encompass speedy onset of movement (with the useful resource of way ofweeks) and better charges of disorder interest score (DAS) remission, which also can in difficulty be due to direct results of IL-6 on acute segment reactants collectively with C-reactive protein. Its critical dangers encompass commonplace liver feature check (LFT) abnormalities, quick neutropenia (even though now not temporally associated with infections), and multiplied levels of cholesterol (requiring statin use in five%). A recent take a look at showed that tocilizumab is rather powerful in a setting near real-lifestyles health center remedy with a speedy and sustained development in symptoms and signs and symptoms and symptoms and signs and signs of RA, and a ability safety profile was visible over the 24-week study length.97 A metanalysis of pooled safety statistics of 4009 sufferers dealt with with tocilizumab over an average period of .4 years said a solid protection profile over time with none new protection indicators.Ninety 8

Rheumatoid Arthritis Treatment Guidelines

American College of Rheumatology

The ACR recommendations for use of artificial DMARDs and biologics within the remedy of RA had been posted in 2008 and up to date in 2012.Eleven,12 The tenet covers caution signs and symptoms to be used, tracking of thing outcomes, the evaluation of scientific responses to DMARDs and biologic sellers, switching among DMARDs and biologic treatments, use of biologics in immoderate-hazard patients (people with hepatitis, congestive coronary coronary heart failure and malignancy, screening for TB in patients beginning or presently receiving biologics, vaccination in sufferers beginning or currently receiving DMARDs or biologics. Medications, which include NSAIDs, and intraarticular and oral corticosteroids, and nonpharmacologic treatment options (together with bodily and occupational treatment alternatives) have been now not included in the hints (the authors advocate that in the destiny, the ACR can also determine to boom broader RA recommendations that encompass remedies that are not in this article). Gold, cyclosporine and azathioprine were not included due to the rare use of these sellers, and the IL-1 receptor antagonist, anakinra have become now not included because of its rare use and lack of recent statistics. Only the ones remedy plans accepted at the time of the literature evaluation are blanketed within the pointers, and embody all criminal biologics defined in this ebook.

The guidelines had been formulated by means of way of a panel of world experts, primarily based on clinical proof coupled with formal organisation system in region of simplest the legal indicators from regulatory groups, and used an frequent confirmed device for developing the tips. For each final recommendation the energy of evidence have become assigned the use of strategies used by the American College of Cardiology99 as follows: A - facts derived from more than one randomized managed medical trials; B - records derived from a single randomized trial or nonrandomized research; and C - statistics derived from consensus opinion of experts, case research, or necessities of care. The authors observe that, regular with the need to extrapolate from scientific revel in in the absence of higher-tier evidence, many new pointers (about seventy nine%) have been associated with diploma C evidence. Furthermore, even though new class requirements for RA (ACR/EULAR) had been published in September 2010,13 the studies evaluated for the 2012 hints trusted the usage of the 1987 ACR RA type criteria10 because of the fact the literature evaluation preceded the ebook of the brand new requirements.

Drawing on statistics and revel in obtained thinking about the truth that 2008 guiding precept, the 2012 recommendations suggest more competitive remedy in early RA because of the expectancy that the earlier the remedy the better the very last outcomes, joint harm is basically irreversible so prevention of damage is crucial, and proof that early considerable remedy may additionally moreover provide the fantastic opportunity to preserve bodily feature and health related exquisite of lifestyles and reduce art work-associated disability.12 The authors assume that in the destiny, data using the modern RA beauty standards may be available for evidence synthesis and formulating hints.

These tips observe to not unusual scientific situations and can not correctly supply all uncertainties and nuances of affected man or woman care in the real worldwide; most effective a clinician's assessment in collaboration with the affected man or woman lets in for the first-rate chance–benefit evaluation on a case-with the aid of manner of-case basis.12

Table four. Summary of American College of Rheumatology (ACR) hints for use of artificial DMARDs and biologics within the treatment of RA (Source: Singh et al. 2012)12

1. Starting, resuming, consisting of, or switching disorder-enhancing anti-rheumatic tablets (DMARDs) or biologic dealers:

1A. Target, both low disorder hobby, or remission for all patients with early rheumatoid arthritis (RA) and hooked up RA, receiving any DMARD or biologic agent.

1B. DMARD monotherapy is usually recommended for early RA (infection duration <6 months) of low sickness interest, or mild or excessive ailment hobby inside the absence of terrible prognostic capabilities. In sufferers with DMARD combination remedy (collectively with double and triple treatment) is usually encouraged for early RA of moderate or excessive illness interest plus terrible prognostic abilties. Additionally, for patients with early RA Anti tumor necrosis element (TNF) biologic without or with methotrexate (MTX) is suggested (infliximab handiest in combination with MTX) for immoderate disease hobby with awful prognostic capabilities.

www.ingramcontent.com/pod-product-compliance
Lightning Source LLC
Chambersburg PA
CBHW060223030426
42335CB00014B/1319